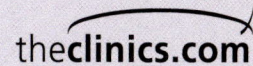

CLINICS IN PLASTIC SURGERY

Evidence-Based Plastic Surgery: Design, Measurement, and Evaluation

Guest Editor
ACHILLEAS THOMA, MD, MSc, FRCS(C), FACS

April 2008 • Volume 35 • Number 2

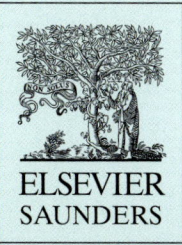

ELSEVIER
SAUNDERS

An imprint of Elsevier, Inc
PHILADELPHIA   LONDON   TORONTO   MONTREAL   SYDNEY   TOKYO

W.B. SAUNDERS COMPANY
A Division of Elsevier Inc.

1600 John F. Kennedy Blvd., Suite 1800, Philadelphia, PA 19103-2899

http://www.theclinics.com

CLINICS IN PLASTIC SURGERY Volume 35, Number 2
April 2008 ISSN 0094-1298, ISBN-13: 978-1-4160-5868-7, ISBN-10: 1-4160-5868-0

Editor: Barbara Cohen-Kligerman

Copyright © 2008 Elsevier Inc. All rights reserved. No part of this publication may be reproduced or transmitted in any form or by any means, electronic or mechanical, including photocopy, recording, or any information retrieval system, without written permission from the publisher.

Single photocopies of single articles may be made for personal use as allowed by national copyright laws. Permission of the publisher and payment of a fee is required for all other photocopying, including multiple or systematic copying, copying for advertising or promotional purposes, resale, and all forms of document delivery. Special rates are available for educational institutions that wish to make photocopies for non-profit educational classroom use. Permissions may be sought directly from Elsevier's Global Rights Department in Oxford, UK: phone 215-239-3804 or +44 (0)1865 843830, fax +44 (0)1865 853333, e-mail: healthpermissions@elsevier.com. Requests may also be completed on-line via the Elsevier homepage (http://www.elsevier.com/permissions). In the USA, users may clear permissions and make payments through the Copyright Clearance Center, Inc., 222 Rosewood Drive, Danvers, MA 01923, USA; phone: (978) 750-8400, fax: (978) 750-4744, and in the UK through the Copyright Licensing Agency Rapid Clearance Service (CLARCS), 90 Tottenham Court Road, London W1P 0LP, UK; phone: (+44) 171 436 5931; fax: (+44) 171 436 3986. Other countries may have a local reprographic rights agency for payments.

Reprints. For copies of 100 or more, of articles in this publication, please contact the Commercial Reprints Department, Elsevier Inc., 360 Park Avenue South, New York, New York 10010-1710. Tel.: (212) 633-3813 Fax: (212) 462-1935, e-mail: reprints@elsevier.com.

The ideas and opinions expressed in *Clinics in Plastic Surgery* do not necessarily reflect those of the Publisher. The Publisher does not assume any responsibility for any injury and/or damage to persons or property arising out of or related to any use of the material contained in this periodical. The reader is advised to check the appropriate medical literature and the product information currently provided by the manufacturer of each drug to be administered to verify the dosage, the method and duration of administration, or contraindications. It is the responsibility of the treating physician or other health care professional, relying on independent experience and knowledge of the patient, to determine drug dosages and the best treatment for the patient. Mention of any product in this issue should not be construed as endorsement by the contributors, editors, or the Publisher of the product or manufacturers' claims.

Clinics in Plastic Surgery (ISSN 0094-1298) is published quarterly by Elsevier Inc., 360 Park Avenue South, New York, NY 10010-1710. Months of issue are January, April, July, and October. Business and Editorial Offices: 1600 John F. Kennedy Blvd., Suite 1800, Philadelphia, PA 19103-2899. Customer Service Office: 6277 Sea Harbor Drive, Orlando, FL 32887-4800. Periodicals postage paid at New York, NY and additional mailing offices. Subscription prices are $326.00 per year for US individuals, $472.00 per year for US institutions, $164.00 per year for US students and residents, $370.00 per year for Canadian individuals, $539.00 per year for Canadian institutions, $395.00 per year for international individuals, $539.00 per year for international institutions, and $195.00 per year for Canadian and foreign students/residents. To receive student/resident rate, orders must be accompanied by name of affiliated institution, date of term, and the *signature* of program/residency coordinator on institution letterhead. Orders will be billed at individual rate until proof of status is received. Foreign air speed delivery is included in all *Clinics* subscription prices. All prices are subject to change without notice.
POSTMASTER: Send address changes to *Clinics in Plastic Surgery*, Elsevier Periodicals Customer Service, 6277 Sea Harbor Drive, Orlando, FL 32887-4800. **Customer Service: 1-800-654-2452 (US). From outside of the US, call 1-407-563-6020. Fax: 1-407-363-9661.**
E-mail: JournalsCustomerService-usa@elsevier.com

Clinics in Plastic Surgery is covered in *Current Contents*, *EMBASE/Excerpta Medica*, *Science Citation Index*, *Index Medicus*, *ASCA*, and *ISI/BIOMED*.

Printed in the United States of America.

EVIDENCE-BASED PLASTIC SURGERY: DESIGN, MEASUREMENT, AND EVALUATION

GUEST EDITOR

ACHILLEAS THOMA, MD, MSc, FRCS(C), FACS
Head and Program Director, Division of Plastic Surgery; Clinical Professor, Department of Surgery; Associate Member, Department of Clinical Epidemiology and Biostatistics; Surgical Outcomes Research Centre (SOURCE), McMaster University, Hamilton, Ontario, Canada

CONTRIBUTORS

AMY K. ALDERMAN, MD, MPH
Assistant Professor of Surgery, Plastic and Reconstructive Surgery, Department of Surgery, University of Michigan, The University of Michigan Medical Center, Ann Arbor, Michigan

MARTIN M. ANTONY, PhD, ABPP
Professor, Department of Psychology, Ryerson University, Toronto, Ontario, Canada

STUART ARCHIBALD, MD, FRCSC, FACS
Associate Professor, Department of Surgery; Head, Division of Otolaryngology–Head and Neck Surgery, St. Joseph's Healthcare, McMaster University, Hamilton, Ontario, Canada

STEFAN J. CANO, PhD
Neurological Outcomes Measures Unit, Institute of Neurology, University College London, London, United Kingdom

SHIM CHING, MSc, MD, FRCSC, FACS
Assistant Clinical Professor, Department of Surgery, University of Hawaii, Honolulu, Hawaii

KEVIN C. CHUNG, MD, MS
Professor of Surgery, Plastic and Reconstructive Surgery, Department of Surgery, University of Michigan, The University of Michigan Medical Center, Ann Arbor, Michigan

ERIC DUKU, MSc, PStat
Senior Statistician, Department of Psychiatry and Behavioural Neurosciences, Offord Centre for Child Studies, McMaster University, Hamilton, Ontario, Canada

CHARLIE H. GOLDSMITH, BSc, MSc, PhD
Emeritus Professor of Biostatistics, Department of Clinical Epidemiology and Biostatistics; Member, Surgical Outcomes Research Centre (SOURCE), McMaster University; and Senior Biostatistician, Biostatistics Unit, St Joseph's Healthcare Hamilton, Hamilton, Ontario, Canada

TED HAINES, MD, MSc, FRCPC
Associate Professor, Department of Clinical Epidemiology and Biostatistics, McMaster University, Hamilton, Ontario, Canada

CAROLYN L. KERRIGAN, MD
Professor of Surgery; Chief and Residency Program Director, Section of Plastic Surgery, Dartmouth-Hitchcock Medical Center, Lebanon, New Hampshire

ANNE F. KLASSEN, DPhil
Associate Professor, Department of Pediatrics, McMaster University, Hamilton, Ontario, Canada

CAROLYN LEVIS, MD, MSc, FRCSC
Assistant Professor, Department of Surgery, Division of Plastic and Reconstructive Surgery, St. Joseph's Healthcare, McMaster University, Hamilton, Ontario, Canada

COLLEEN McCARTHY, MD, MSc
Memorial Sloan-Kettering Cancer Center, New York, New York

PAULA McKAY, BSc
Research Coordinator, Department of Surgery, McMaster University, Hamilton, Ontario, Canada

LESLIE McKNIGHT, MSc
Research Assistant, Department of Surgery, Division of Plastic Surgery, McMaster University, Hamilton, Ontario, Canada

FRANK PAPANIKOLAOU, MD, FRCSC
Urological Surgeon, Mississauga, Ontario, Canada

LENORA PERRY, BSc
Research Assistant, Department of Clinical Epidemiology and Biostatistics, McMaster University, Hamilton; and Department of Medicine, University of Western Ontario, London Health Sciences Centre, London, Ontario, Canada

ANDREA L. PUSIC, MD, MHS
Assistant Professor, Plastic and Reconstructive Surgery, Memorial Sloan-Kettering Cancer Center, New York, New York

GLORIA ROCKWELL, MD, MSc, FRCSC
Assistant Professor, Department of Surgery, Division of Plastic Surgery, University of Ottawa, Ottawa, Ontario, Canada

ERIK D. SKARSGARD, MD
Associate Professor, Department of Surgery (Pediatric General Surgery), University of British Columbia, Vancouver, British Columbia, Canada

SHEILA SPRAGUE, MSc
Senior Research Coordinator, Department of Clinical Epidemiology and Biostatistics, McMaster University, Hamilton, Ontario, Canada

MITCHELL A. STOTLAND, MD
Associate Professor of Surgery (Pediatric) and Pediatrics; and Director, Craniofacial Anomalies Clinic, Dartmouth-Hitchcock Medical Center, Lebanon, New Hampshire

NICK STRUMAS, MD, FRCSC
Assistant Professor, Department of Surgery, Division of Plastic and Reconstructive Surgery, McMaster University, Hamilton, Ontario, Canada

CLAIRE TEMPLE, MD, FRCSC
Department of Surgery, Division of Plastic and Reconstructive Surgery, University of Western Ontario, Hand and Upper Limb Centre, London, Ontario, Canada

ACHILLEAS THOMA, MD, MSc, FRCS(C), FACS
Head and Program Director, Division of Plastic Surgery; Clinical Professor, Department of Surgery; Associate Member, Department of Clinical Epidemiology and Biostatistics; Surgical Outcomes Research Centre (SOURCE), McMaster University, Hamilton, Ontario, Canada

EVIDENCE-BASED PLASTIC SURGERY: DESIGN, MEASUREMENT, AND EVALUATION

Contents

Preface
Achilleas Thoma

Forming the Research Question   189
Achilleas Thoma, Leslie McKnight, Paula McKay, and Ted Haines

The most important precondition for performing a clinical research project in plastic surgery, or any other surgical subspecialty, is the need to ask the "right question." Although this might seem to be an easy task, in truth it requires a lot of effort and hard work. This article addresses the key points to remember when formulating a research question.

Study Design and Hierarchy of Evidence for Surgical Decision Making   195
Sheila Sprague, Paula McKay, and Achilleas Thoma

This article provides a historical overview of the hierarchy of evidence for surgical decision making and discusses key study designs in the hierarchy of evidence. This encompasses meta-analyses, randomized controlled trials, and observational studies, including cohort and case-controlled studies, case series and case reports, and basic science studies. This article also reviews the principles and importance of evidence-based plastic surgery and describes several systems to rate the strength of the scientific evidence.

The Role of Systematic Reviews in Clinical Research and Practice   207
Ted Haines, Leslie McKnight, Eric Duku, Lenora Perry, and Achilleas Thoma

Well-conducted systematic reviews and meta-analyses provide the best quality evidence for clinical decision-making. This article presents the key role of systematic reviews in clinical decision-making, discussing the steps and pitfalls to avoid in conducting systematic reviews and meta-analyses.

Clinical Research in Breast Surgery: Reduction and Postmastectomy Reconstruction 215
Andrea L. Pusic, Colleen McCarthy, Stefan J. Cano, Anne F. Klassen, and Carolyn L. Kerrigan

In the last decade, entirely new techniques in breast reduction and reconstruction have evolved. What remains unclear is whether or not these new procedures, some of which carry additional surgical risk and cost, are superior from a patient perspective. Thus, plastic surgeons are ever more reliant on clinical research to provide high-level evidence to facilitate clinical decision-making, as well as policy negotiations and advocacy. This article provides an overview of the strengths and weaknesses of different study designs, the appropriateness of various outcome measures, and the importance of establishing a strong evidence base in breast surgery.

Clinical Research in Head and Neck Reconstruction 227
Carolyn Levis and Stuart Archibald

Reconstructive head and neck surgery is not unlike other surgical fields in its paucity of clinical research. Difficulties exist in the design and execution of surgical studies, and there are many challenges and limitations that must be addressed. In this article, the types of studies that make up head and neck reconstructive literature are reviewed, as well as the evolution toward the use of quality-of-life scales, which measure patients' satisfaction with their state of health and function.

Measuring Outcomes in Hand Surgery 239
Amy K. Alderman and Kevin C. Chung

Outcomes research in hand surgery provides patients and providers with objective, reliable information to assist in making medical decisions. Endpoint measures in outcomes research and the instruments used to evaluate these endpoints are often specific to a particular disease or region. Hand surgery has many different measurable outcomes that can be used to monitor the quality of surgical practice, inform practice guidelines, and aid in the appropriate allocation of healthcare resources. In this article, we review some research techniques available to study the following surgical outcomes of the hand: national trends in surgical care, surgical complications, objective measures of hand function, patient-reported measures of hand function, and economic burden.

Clinical Research in Pediatric Plastic Surgery and Systematic Review of Quality-of-Life Questionnaires 251
Anne F. Klassen, Mitchell A. Stotland, Erik D. Skarsgard, and Andrea L. Pusic

In the first part of this article, examples of different research designs used to study pediatric patients who undergo plastic surgery are described. The remainder of the article discusses the measurement of outcomes in pediatric plastic surgery research, with a particular focus on the assessment of quality of life (QOL). Issues specific to measuring QOL in children are discussed (eg, developmental considerations, use of self- versus proxy report). The results of a systematic literature review to identify and appraise pediatric plastic surgery condition-specific measures of QOL are presented.

Clinical Research in Aesthetic Surgery 269
Shim Ching, Gloria Rockwell, Achilleas Thoma, and Martin M. Antony

Clinical research in aesthetic surgery cannot use traditional objective measures of surgical success. Present research designs and methods used in aesthetic surgery limit the ability to conduct meaningful clinical research. Outcomes research may be ideally suited for assessing patients in aesthetic surgery. A critical aspect of an outcomes-based approach is to select appropriate instruments for investigations. Widely accepted, standardized methods for assessing outcomes would allow for comparison of surgical techniques and provide a common basis for clinical investigations.

The Role of the Randomized Controlled Trial in Plastic Surgery 275
Achilleas Thoma, Sheila Sprague, Claire Temple, and Stuart Archibald

This article discusses the role of the randomized controlled trial (RCT) in plastic surgery. There are unique challenges in the execution of an RCT in plastic surgery, including: (1) surgical equipoise, (2) the surgical learning curve, (3) differential care, (4) randomization, (5) concealment, (6) expertise-based design, (7) blinding, (8) intention-to-treat analysis, (9) loss to follow-up, and (10) treatment effect and implications for sample size calculations. The RCTs conducted in plastic surgery to date are generally of poor quality in design and reporting, are fraught with bias, and have small sample sizes, thus this article attempts to help future investigators perform better quality RCTs.

The Use of Cost-effectiveness Analysis in Plastic Surgery Clinical Research 285
Achilleas Thoma, Nick Strumas, Gloria Rockwell, and Leslie McKnight

The goal of this article is to introduce clinical investigators to the basic concepts of cost-effectiveness analysis. This line of research is not commonly pursued in clinical studies probably because of unfamiliarity of plastic surgeons with the field of health economics and health research methodology in general. The authors believe that the coupling of cost-effectiveness analysis with clinical studies is important and should be incorporated into surgical clinical research.

Testing Quality Improvement Interventions 297
Frank Papanikolaou and Charlie H. Goldsmith

The quality of health care is in drastic need of improvement. Surgeons are key players in the health care delivery system, and as such, they should be involved by leading or participating in the improvements that should take place. This article posits some suggestions as to how surgeons can participate in the efforts to make the health care provided to patients better and make the system a better place to work for surgeons and for other health professionals. Participation in quality improvement (QI) initiatives has the potential to bring much personal satisfaction for surgeons who help the process to move forward, even though it takes some effort and even forces them to learn some new skills and attitudes to what can be accomplished by QI teams. This article provides a methodologic guide to conducting and evaluating QI research.

How to Become a Successful Clinical Investigator 305
Achilleas Thoma, Ted Haines, Eric Duku, Leslie McKnight, and Charlie Goldsmith

The purpose of this article is to help residents, fellows, and junior faculty who aspire to an academic career, and seasoned plastic surgeons who may wish to have a second research-oriented "lease on life," to become successful clinical investigators. The preconditions for academic success, including mentoring, making periodic priority lists, and time management are discussed in detail.

Index 313

FORTHCOMING ISSUES

July 2008
Facelifts, Part I
Malcolm D. Paul, MD, *Guest Editor*

October 2008
Facelifts, Part II
Malcolm D. Paul, MD, *Guest Editor*

January 2009
Breast Augmentation
Scott L. Spear, MD, *Guest Editor*

RECENT ISSUES

January 2008
Body Contouring After Massive Weight Loss
Al Aly, MD, FACS, *Guest Editor*

October 2007
Wound Surgery
Mark S. Granick, MD, FACS, *Guest Editor*

July 2007
Orthognathic Surgery
Pravin K. Patel, MD, *Guest Editor*

THE CLINICS ARE NOW AVAILABLE ONLINE!

Access your subscription at:
www.theclinics.com

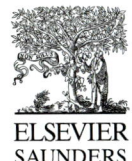

Preface

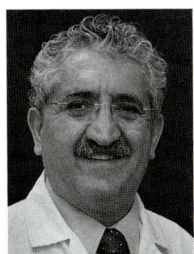

Achilleas Thoma, MD, MSc, FRCS(C), FACS
Guest Editor

Achilleas Thoma, MD, MSc, FRCS(C), FACS*
Department of Surgery, Division of Plastic Surgery;
Department of Clinical Epidemiology and Biostatistics;
Surgical Outcomes Research Centre (SOURCE);
McMaster University, Hamilton, Ontario, Canada

E-mail address:
athoma@mcmaster.ca

Plastic surgeons strive to offer their patients the surgical techniques and procedures that maximize benefit and minimize harm. Many different factors influence clinical decisions, including the clinical state of the patient, the clinical setting, the circumstances under which the surgeon is working, patients' preferences, and the clinician's expertise. Central to the decision-making process however, should be the best research evidence.

Evidence-based plastic surgery integrates the best research evidence with clinical expertise and patient values. In contrast to the traditional approach to plastic surgery practice, the evidence-based approach acknowledges that intuition, "hunches," unsystematic clinical experience, and evidence from the basic science laboratory are insufficient grounds for clinical decision making.

The purpose of this issue is to help surgeons at any stage in their careers, from residents and clinical fellows to established clinical surgeons and academic practitioners, address important clinical questions through correct research methods. Although the issue is targeted primarily at the plastic surgical community, other surgical subspecialties can benefit from it, because most of the concepts covered here are applicable to surgery in general.

This issue discusses many scientific principles and strategies that will help answer important clinical questions in surgery through properly designed studies.

The articles have been arranged in a specific order to guide the reader: (1) How to formulate clinically important questions; (2) What study design can best answer the research question; (3) How to measure the results of surgical interventions, in particular the health status and quality of life of patients; (4) How to evaluate one's work through cost-effectiveness analysis; and, finally, (5) How to become a successful clinical investigator.

Because most jurisdictions have finite health care resources, one of the articles emphasizes the importance of performing cost-effectiveness analysis alongside randomized, controlled trials. We consider this study design the best in the hierarchy of evidence for clinical decisions, and we encourage clinical researchers to adopt it.

*Correspondence. 206 James Street South, Suite 101, Hamilton, ON L8P 3A9, Canada

The credibility of the surgical specialties is contingent on evidence provided by methodologically sound clinical research. It is hoped that this issue of *Clinics in Plastic Surgery* will help the readers in this regard and assist them in coming closer to the "elusive" truth.

It has been my honor to edit this issue of *Clinics in Plastic Surgery*. All the contributors have expertise in health research methodology or public health. I thank them all for their enthusiasm for this project. I also thank Ms. Sarah Barth, Publisher, and Elsevier for their help in this endeavor.

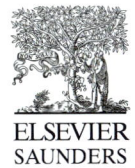

Forming the Research Question

Achilleas Thoma, MD, MSc, FRCS(C), FACS[a,b,c,*], Leslie McKnight, MSc[b], Paula McKay, BSc[d], Ted Haines, MD, MSc, FRCPC[a]

- Identifying clinically relevant questions
- Initial groundwork for research question formulation
- *Plausibility*
- *Feasibility of the research design*
- Support
- Resources
- Formulating the final research question
- Summary
- References

In clinical practice, when doing rounds with residents, or in academic rounds, journal clubs, or clinical conferences, questions are frequently raised for which clinicians don't know the answer. If a literature search of various electronic databases does not provide the answer, and the question is believed to be clinically important, this may be the impetus for a research project. Some of you who are working in academic centers may encourage your resident or fellow to pursue a research project and find the answer to this question. However, the support provided to the resident or fellow may be variable, depending on your own circumstances. It can vary from minimal to exemplary support from a well-defined, organized research team that provides biostatistical and methodologic support. If the support is minimal, it is highly unlikely this research will lead to meaningful results. On the other hand, support within "a well greased research group" makes it more likely that the effort will lead to meaningful findings and culminate in one or more publications.

(See the article by Thoma, Haines, Duku, McKnight, and Goldsmith in this issue.)

The most important precondition for performing a clinical research project in plastic surgery (or any other surgical subspecialty) is the need to ask the "right question." Although this might seem to be an easy task, in truth it requires a lot of effort and hard work. It may take up to a year or more before a clear research question emerges. However, when the question is finally formulated, much of the work entailed in the project has already been done.

Identifying clinically relevant questions

Before beginning a research project, it is important to consider what types of questions are worth addressing. Investigators undertake a research question because they are not happy with the outcomes of a particular surgical intervention or approach to a clinical problem. The intervention question should be of importance to the patients

---

[a] Department of Clinical Epidemiology and Biostatistics, McMaster University, Hamilton Health Sciences Centre, 1200 Main Street West, Hamilton, ON L8N 3Z5, Canada
[b] Department of Surgery, Division of Plastic Surgery, McMaster University, St. Joseph's Healthcare, 50 Charlton Avenue East, Hamilton, ON L8N 4A6, Canada
[c] Surgical Outcomes Research Centre (SOURCE), McMaster University, St. Joseph's Healthcare, 50 Charlton Avenue East, Hamilton, ON L8N 4A6, Canada
[d] Department of Surgery, McMaster University, 293 Wellington Street North, Suite 110, Hamilton, ON L8L 8E7, Canada
* Corresponding author. 206 James Street South, Suite 101, Hamilton, ON L8P 3A9, Canada.
E-mail address: athoma@mcmaster.ca (A. Thoma).

because it may improve pain or ability to return to gainful employment, or improve their quality of life overall. Questions that need to be addressed are ones that are clinically relevant (Box 1).

Research questions may lead to solutions to clinically important problems because, from the societal perspective, current surgical interventions consume significant health care resources. Even if they do not consume significant resources singly, if they are very common, cumulatively they may do so. For example, a hand transplant may consume large health care resources, but if it is performed infrequently, then it will be of no great consequence to the society. On the other hand, hand transplantation costs at the societal level may be dwarfed by a procedure that is less expensive at the level of the individual case, such as an endoscopic carpal tunnel release (ECTR), which because of its frequency cumulatively may cost more to the society. Therefore, a research question on the effectiveness of ECTR, rather than hand transplantation, may be more appropriate in terms of societal impact. Questions that do not address a significant burden in terms of cost, prevalence, or severity should not be considered as the motivation for clinical research activity, as they consume time, energy, and resources which could be expended more efficiently in worthwhile projects. This decision, however, requires judgment and may even require expert consensus. In other words, the difference between a clinically important question and a trivial one may not be apparent to a novice investigator. The pursuit of scholarship, a mentorship period, or an attachment to a research group will enable a young investigator to learn how to ask the important questions.

To formulate a proper clinical research question, the investigator (who may be a surgical resident, fellow, or surgeon) must have extensive knowledge of the subject matter he or she is investigating. In other words, he or she "must know the boundary between current knowledge and ignorance" [1]. The researchable question comes from finding the "cutting edge" of knowledge for a health problem you are familiar with [1]. Before embarking on the research project, it is important to summarize this "cutting edge evidence" in the form of a systematic review (see the article by Haines, McKnight, Duku, Perry, and Thoma in this issue).

For example, one clinical question that arose in the authors' surgical group was whether ECTR was more effective than open carpal tunnel release (OCTR) for the treatment of carpal tunnel syndrome. Although the authors were performing both techniques in our clinical practice, we were uncertain that ECTR was more effective than OCTR. To formulate the research question, we performed an extensive literature search on the subject and familiarized ourselves with the current evidence. Only when we thought we had found the "cutting edge" of knowledge on the subject did we then feel comfortable developing our research question [2]. This scholarship allowed us to carry out a research project, in this case a meta-analysis, designed to determine whether ECTR was more effective than OCTR [3]. The findings from one research project may lead to other questions as well, providing the basis for further research. In the case of ECTR, we wanted to know if this novel technique was a cost-effective procedure, leading us to an economic evaluation of ECTR versus OCTR [4].

Initial groundwork for research question formulation

Before beginning the process of explicit formulation of the research question, it is important to consider several factors, bearing on whether the project will be practicable [5]. These include: (1) the plausibility of the question (whether or not it is answerable); (2) the feasibility of the proposed design to answer the question; (3) the support you expect to obtain from your surgical colleagues; and (4) the resources available to you.

Plausibility

When evaluating the plausibility of a research question, it is important to consider whether or not the question is answerable. To determine plausibility, one must have a thorough understanding of the anatomy, biology, physiology, and prevalence of the problem. In short, the question being asked should be within the realm of the plastic surgeon's expertise. For example, it would not be plausible for a clinical investigator to examine the outcomes of reconstruction of the congenitally absent ear in a parallel randomized controlled trial (RCT) comparing the Nagata technique [6,7] with the genetic engineering method, because the genetic engineering methods are not advanced enough at this point in time to regenerate an acceptable ear.

Box 1: Reasons to pursue a clinical research question

- The intervention is novel
- The intervention consumes large health care resources
- There is a controversy on the effectiveness of the novel procedure (as compared with the existing procedure)
- There is a large cost difference between two prevailing interventions

Feasibility of the research design

Evaluating the feasibility of a question involves determining whether the study design chosen is one that can potentially answer the research question. There is no such thing as one best study design; the best study design will depend on what the question is. For example, it would be fruitless to attempt to answer the question of whether smoking affects the short-term survival of replanted digits with an RCT design. The main barrier to using this design is that smoking is a harmful activity. Ethically, investigators cannot randomize patients to either Group A: continue smoking, or Group B: non-smoking after replantation of digits. For questions of harm, appropriate study designs include case-controlled studies and cohort studies (see the article by Sprague, McKay, and Thoma in this issue).

Another example of a hypothetical research question that may not be feasible to answer is whether the supramicrosurgical reconstruction with a periumbilical abdominal flap is superior to the deep inferior epigastric perforator flap in breast reconstruction [8]. Possible barriers to answering this research question could be: the investigators don't know how to transfer a flap with a 0.8-mm luminal diameter of the vascular pedicle; the investigators don't have the required delicate instruments to perform the supramicrosurgery; and the quality-of-life scales that are available may not be sensitive enough to capture the differential effect of the competing interventions.

Another example raising issues of feasibility would be a project in which a clinical investigator intends to perform an RCT comparing the use of intermittent lower extremity pump versus low molecular heparin in preventing fatal pulmonary embolism in cosmetic abdominoplasty. Fatal pulmonary embolism in cosmetic abdominoplasty is a very rare event. As the frequency of the "end points" is a critical factor in the sample size calculation, the rarity of the target event means that the investigator will require a sample size measured in thousands of patients, making it unlikely that he or she will be able to answer the proposed question.

Most clinical research is incremental in nature. The more research that has been done previously, the more investigators can do presently. If there are big gaps in knowledge, it may be prudent to start with a simpler and less expensive study design, such as a case series or cohort study (lower level of evidence), and advance from there. The appropriate time to perform an RCT (higher level of evidence) comparing two surgical interventions is when a novel surgical intervention has entered the main stream of surgery and challenges a prevailing one (see the article by Thoma, Sprague, Temple, and Archibald in this issue).

Support

The support we expect from our colleagues is another important consideration when evaluating a proposed research question. Because most plastic surgeons are unlikely to have a sufficient number of patients with the condition of interest to meet the sample size requirements, investigators frequently rely on their colleagues to contribute cases. We may tempt them by making them collaborators in research design and interpretation and coauthors in future publication. Unfortunately, many plastic surgeons are entrenched into their beliefs that their preferred technique is the only one that works. For example, in the authors' division, we encountered resistance in persuading some of our colleagues to participate in an RCT comparing intramuscular versus submuscular transposition of the ulnar nerve at the level of the elbow after electromyography-proven clinical entrapment neuropathy of the ulnar nerve. While initially enthusiastic about participating in the study, some of them were subsequently unwilling to submit their patients to randomization.

Resources

The financial resources available for the project are also crucial to the ultimate completion of the study. It is important that a realistic budget be considered, and that the study commence only after funding from local or peer-reviewed grant competitions has been secured. It would be a mistake to commence the project without the funds required to meet its ongoing needs, such as support for a study coordinator.

Formulating the final research question

When formulating the final research question, the investigator should, in general, aim to ask a "foreground" question as compared with a "background" question. Background questions have three essential components: a question root (who, what, where, when, how, why) together with a verb and a disorder, or an aspect of a disorder of interest [9]. For example, a background question would be: "what complications can occur with the free transverse rectus abdominis musculocutaneous (TRAM) flap?" or "why does the TRAM sometimes suffer necrosis?" These types of questions seek to increase basic or background understanding about the disorder of interest.

Foreground questions, on the other hand, are more directly applicable to practice, because they ask specifically how to manage patients. To formulate the final, well-constructed clinical question, five elements, often captured by the acronym PICOT, need to be incorporated [10].

P: Describe the Population or Patients relevant to the question
I: Define the surgical Intervention
C: Define the Comparative intervention
O: Describe the Outcomes of interest, and
T: Define the Time horizon for measurement of the outcome.

When defining these elements of PICOT, it is important to be specific. The population should briefly and precisely describe a specific group of patients. Basically, the investigator is asking, "How can I describe a group of patients similar to mine?" For example, in a research project on carpal tunnel release, an investigator may consider excluding only patients with handwork exposure, or may decide to allocate them to a subgroup of the study.

When defining the intervention, the investigator must determine the main intervention, prognostic factor, or exposure he or she is interested in. For example, the investigator may be interested in the effectiveness of the ECTR versus OCTR. As there are many variations of the ECTR release, the investigator needs to be specific about which one he intends to use. For example he may decide to consider the Agee and colleagues [11] endoscopic carpal tunnel release and not the Chow technique [12]. The comparison is then defined as the main alternative to the intervention. In the case of a surgical intervention, this may be an alternative surgical technique or perhaps conservative management.

The comparative intervention to the ECTR may be the OCTR. Here there are various techniques, such as the classical approach, with a long incision from the wrist crease to the proximal palmar crease or very small incisions over the carpal tunnel area (1 cm–2 cm). Again, the investigator needs to specify which of these variations he or she is using.

When defining "outcomes," investigators are asking, "What can I hope to accomplish, measure, improve, or affect?" For any given plastic surgery problem, there are numerous clinically relevant outcomes. Therefore, it is important to be specific when selecting which outcomes are relevant to the question. For example, when considering the outcomes of carpal tunnel release, the investigator may be interested in return to work of specific ergonomic characteristics, return to activities of daily living, pain control, or adjusted quality-of-life years. The choice of outcome measures should consider the relevant perspectives of, for example, surgeon, patient, society, hospital, or primary payer. The surgeon may consider a successful flap as the primary outcome measure, whereas the patient would consider improvement in quality of life an important outcome. It is important to consider all outcomes relevant to the intervention, from as many perspectives as feasible (see the article by Thoma, Strumas, Rockwell, and McKnight in this issue).

Time horizon refers to the most appropriate time to measure the outcome of interest. The outcomes may be associated with different time horizons, and the time horizons require consideration of whether the investigator is interested in short, intermediate, or long-term follow-ups. For example, a digital replant may be a success at the short follow-up of 3 weeks in terms of survival, but at the long-term follow-up, it may be considered a failure if the digit becomes nonsensate and stiff, and hinders the patient from returning to work at a year's time. There should be consensus among the research team as to when a particular outcome should be measured.

Recently, the authors' research group wanted to determine whether the superficial inferior epigastric artery flap was more cost-effective than the deep inferior epigastric perforator flap in postmastectomy reconstruction. For this investigation, the essential elements of the question were as follows:

P: The population of interest was all patients who underwent postmastectomy reconstruction
I: The surgical intervention being studied was the superficial inferior epigastric artery flap
C: The comparative surgical intervention was the deep inferior epigastric perforator flap
O: The outcomes of interest were cost-effectiveness and health-related quality of life
T: The time horizon was the patient's remaining life

This yielded the following research question: *In postmastectomy patients undergoing reconstruction, is the superficial inferior epigastric artery flap more cost-effective than the deep inferior epigastric perforator flap?*

The research question guides the literature search, protocol development, and conduct of the study. Thus, a well-defined question will serve as a reference point throughout the study. However, the research question is but one aspect of a larger iterative process. This iterative process is shown in **Fig. 1** [13].

There is a tendency among clinical investigators to ask multiple questions in a clinical study. It is important to understand that all the primary and secondary questions need to be asked up front. This ensures that the questions are hypothesis driven (ie, based on predictions of what will happen) rather than data driven (ie, made up after the study results are in, especially to explain findings that may well be simply the play of chance) [1].

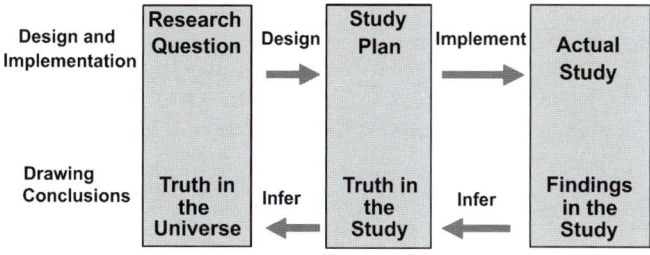

Fig. 1. The iterative research process. (*From* Hulley SB, Cummings SR, Browner WS, et al. Designing Clinical Research, 2nd Edition. Philadelphia: Lippincott Williams & Wilkins, 2001; with permission.)

The crucial distinction between the primary and the secondary questions is that only the primary question will be able to provide a definitive answer. This is because the sample size of the study will be based only on the primary questions. Any answers obtained from the secondary questions need to be considered as tenuous or hypothesis generating. They may need to be addressed in another study, in which they become the primary questions. The authors' recommendation is to simplify the surgical research project and consider relying on only one well-developed primary question.

Summary

The key points to remember when formulating the research question are:

1. Focus on a single primary research question; this will determine the calculation of the sample size of the study (see the article by Thoma, Sprague, Temple, and Archibald in this issue).
2. Develop the primary research question in a structured manner (PICOT formulation).
3. Perform a systematic review to reach the "boundary of knowledge" on the subject you are investigating (see the article by Haines, McKnight, Duku, Perry, and Thoma in this issue).
4. Gain an understanding of clinical research methodology, find a mentor, and preferably work within a research group (see the article by Thoma, Haines, Duku, McKnight, and Goldsmith in this issue).
5. Ensure that a biostatistician is involved early on in the formulation of the question and the execution of the study.

References

[1] Haynes RB, Sackett DL, Guyatt GH, et al. Clinical epidemiology: how to do clinical practice research. 3rd edition. Philadelphia: Lippincott Williams & Wilkins; 2006.

[2] Thoma A, Veltri K, Haines T, et al. A systematic review of reviews comparing endoscopic and open carpal tunnel decompression. Plast Reconstr Surg 2004;13:1184–91.

[3] Thoma A, Veltri K, Haines T, et al. A meta-analysis of RCTs comparing endoscopic and open CT decompression. Plast Reconstr Surg 2004;114:1137–45.

[4] Thoma A, Wong VH, Sprague S, et al. A cost-utility analysis of open and endoscopic carpal tunnel release. Canadian Journal of Plastic Surgery 2006;15:15–20.

[5] Haynes BR. Forming the research question. J Clin Epidemiol 2006;59:881–6.

[6] Nagata S. Modification of the stages in total reconstruction of the auricle: part I. grafting the three-dimensional costal cartilage framework for lobule-type microtia. Plast Reconstr Surg 1994;93:221–30.

[7] Nagata S. Modification of the stages in total reconstruction of the auricle: part II grafting the three-dimensional costal cartilage framework for conchal-type microtia. Plast Reconstr Surg 1994;93:231–42.

[8] Koshima I, Inagawa K, Yamamoto M, et al. New microsurgical breast reconstruction using free paraumbilical perforator adiposal flaps. Plast Reconstr Surg 2000;106:61–5.

[9] Sackett DL, Straus SE, Richardson WS, et al. Evidence-based medicine: how to practice and teach EBM. 2nd edition. Edinburgh (Scotland): Churchill Livingstone; 2000.

[10] Guyatt G, Rennie D. Users' guides to the Medical Literature: a manual for evidence-based clinical practice. In: Guyatt G, Rennie D, editors. JAMA & Archives Journals. Chicago: American Medical Association; 2002.

[11] Agee JM, McCarroll HR Jr, Tortosa RD, et al. Endoscopic release of the carpal tunnel: a randomized prospective multicenter study. J Hand Surg (Am) 1992;17(6):987–95.

[12] Chow JC. Endoscopic release of the carpal ligament for carpal tunnel syndrome: 22-month clinical result. Arthroscopy 1990;6(4):288–96.

[13] Hulley SB, Cummungs SR, Browner WS, et al. Designing clinical research. 2nd edition. Philadelphia: Lippincott Williams & Wilkins; 2001.

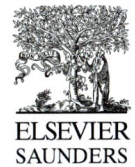

CLINICS IN PLASTIC SURGERY

Study Design and Hierarchy of Evidence for Surgical Decision Making

Sheila Sprague, MSc[a], Paula McKay, BSc[b], Achilleas Thoma, MD, MSc, FRCS(C), FACS[a,c,d,*]

- Historical perspective
- Systematic reviews and meta-analyses
- Randomized controlled trials
- Observational studies: cohort studies and case-controlled studies
- Case reports and series
- Basic science or physiologic studies
- Limitations of using the hierarchy of evidence
- Grading the strength of a body of evidence
- Evidence-based plastic surgery
- Summary
- References

Surgical therapy decisions have historically been based on existing surgical dogma, personal experience, recommendations of surgical authorities, and thoughtful application of surgical basic sciences [1]. As plastic surgeons strive to offer their patients the surgical techniques and procedures that maximize benefit and minimize harm, many different factors may influence their clinical decision-making, including the clinical state of the patient, the clinical setting (academic versus private practices, rural versus urban settings), circumstances (emergency versus elective surgery), patient preferences, and the plastic surgeon's expertise (Fig. 1). The availability of health care resources may also have an impact on surgical decisions; for example, academic centers may have ample technologic resources that are lacking in rural settings, where only basic technology exists.

In addition to these considerations, research evidence also plays a significant role in clinical decisions. It is often challenging to decide which parts of the existing or growing body of clinical research evidence to consider, and how to apply these research findings when making surgical decisions for specific patients. A literature search to address a particular plastic surgery question using an electronic database, such as Medline, may provide a multitude of articles with conflicting recommendations.

The introduction of evidence-based clinical practice [2] in the last two decades has provided direction on how to identify the best available

---

[a] Department of Clinical Epidemiology and Biostatistics, McMaster University, 293 Wellington Street North, Suite 110, Hamilton, ON L8L 8E7, Canada
[b] Department of Surgery, McMaster University, 293 Wellington Street North, Suite 110, Hamilton, Ontario L8L 8E7, Canada
[c] Department of Surgery, Division of Plastic Surgery, McMaster University, St. Joseph's Healthcare, 50 Charlton Avenue East, Hamilton, ON L8N 4A6, Canada
[d] Surgical Outcomes Research Centre (SOURCE), McMaster University, St. Joseph's Healthcare, 50 Charlton Avenue East, Hamilton, ON L8N 4A6, Canada
* Corresponding author. 206 James Street South, Suite 101, Hamilton, ON L8P 3A9, Canada.
E-mail address: athoma@mcmaster.ca (A. Thoma).

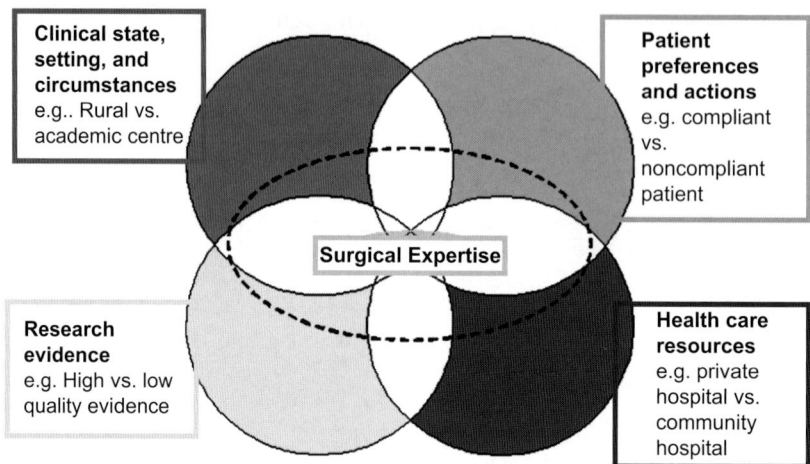

Fig. 1. Factors in making decisions in plastic surgery.

evidence. Evidence-based clinical practice can be defined as the integration of the best research evidence with clinical expertise, while factoring patient values into clinical decision making [2]. In contrast to the traditional approach to plastic surgical practice, the evidence-based plastic surgery approach acknowledges that intuition, unsystematic clinical experience, and pathophysiologic rationale are insufficient grounds for clinical decision-making. It also stresses the importance of examining the evidence from clinical research. It is important for plastic surgeons to apply principles of evidence-based plastic surgery when deciding which of the competing surgical techniques and procedures to use on their patients [3].

Not all research evidence is judged to be of equal value. That is, different research designs have different strengths and, therefore, different levels of value in the decision making process [4]. For surgeons, the integration of research evidence into daily practice requires an understanding of what constitutes high and low quality evidence. Before making a clinical decision, a plastic surgeon must be aware of the strength of the available evidence, and therefore the degree of confidence associated with a decision based on that evidence. The hierarchy of evidence is often represented by a pyramid, in which studies that represent the best evidence are placed at the top, and those representing low quality evidence are placed at the bottom (Fig. 2). When facing a patient with a particular problem, plastic surgeons should seek answers by looking at the best available evidence. For studies evaluating the best surgical treatment in descending order, the authors recommend the following hierarchy of evidence: meta-analysis and systematic reviews of high quality randomized controlled trials, randomized controlled trials, cohort studies, case-controlled studies, case series, expert opinions, and in vitro and animal studies (see Fig. 2). This ranking has an evolutionary order, moving from simple observational methods at the bottom of the pyramid, through to increasingly sophisticated and statistically refined study designs at the top of the pyramid. Unfortunately, many of the publications in the plastic surgery literature fall into the lower levels of the evidence pyramid.

The purpose of this article is to provide a historical overview of the hierarchy of evidence and discuss key study designs in the hierarchy of evidence, including meta-analyses, randomized controlled trials, and observational studies, including cohort studies and case controlled studies, case series and case reports, and basic science studies. Several systems to rate the strength of

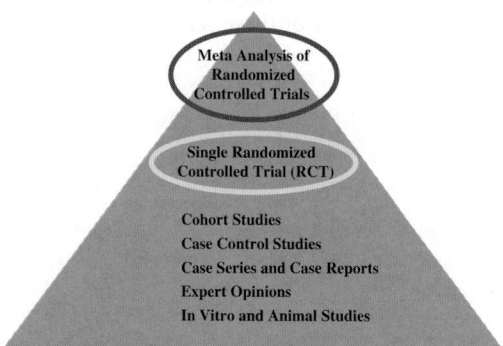

Fig. 2. Hierarchy of evidence pyramid. The meta-analysis of randomized controlled trials (RCT) is considered the best evidence, followed by a large RCT with a narrow confidence interval.

the scientific evidence are described, and some potential limitations of using the hierarchy of evidence are discussed. The principles and importance of evidence-based plastic surgery are also reviewed.

Historical perspective

In the last two decades, there has been an increasing emphasis on basing healthcare and surgical decisions on the best available research evidence. In the late 1970s, the Canadian Task Force on the Periodic Health Examination first popularized hierarchies of evidence, and since that time many different hierarchies have been developed and used [5–9]. Through his book *Effectiveness and Efficiency: Random Reflections on Health Services* (1972) and his subsequent advocacy, Professor Archie Cochrane, a Scottish epidemiologist, fostered an increasing acceptance of the concepts behind evidence-based practice [10]. The explicit methodologies used to determine "best evidence" were largely established by the McMaster University research group, led by Professors David Sackett and Gordon Guyatt. Professors Oxman and Guyatt [11] published the first series on guidelines for reviewing the literature in the Journal of the Canadian Medical Association in the 1980s. The term "evidence-based medicine" first appeared in the medical literature in 1992 in an article by Guyatt and colleagues [2]. In 1993, the *Journal of the American Medical Association* (JAMA) began publishing a series of articles titled the *Users' Guides to the Medical Literature* that described the principles of evidence-based medicine [12]. As the examples provided by the JAMA articles were relevant to medical subspecialties and not easily understood by surgeons, the *Canadian Journal of Surgery* has more recently published a similar series, titled *Users' Guide to the Surgical Literature*, with a surgical spin to make the content more applicable to the surgical community [13]. The intention of these series of articles is to help surgeons discriminate the good from bad articles, based on the methods used and the results reported.

Systematic reviews and meta-analyses

The reviews frequently published in the plastic surgery literature include narrative reviews, systematic reviews, and meta-analyses. A narrative review typically focuses on a broad topic and provides a summary of the literature, but the methods used to locate the literature are not systematic and the included studies are not evaluated on their scientific merits [4]. Narrative reviews may be fraught with bias, as the authors may select articles that espouse their point of view and ignore others that support a contrasting view [4]. This bias can be reduced by conducting a systematic review: a scientific investigation of the literature on a given topic in which the "subjects" are the articles being evaluated [14]. Before a research team conducts a systematic review, a well-designed protocol is developed that includes a focused research question, a specific search strategy, how studies will be identified and selected, inclusion and exclusion criteria, the types of data to be abstracted from each article, and how the data will be synthesized [14]. These key steps are taken to reduce bias in the identification, selection, and use of published work in these reviews [4].

When several RCTs become available, a meta-analysis of these trials provides the highest level of evidence to support a specific treatment [15]. A meta-analysis is a term used for systematic reviews that use quantitative methods or statistical techniques to summarize the results [15]. The aim of a meta-analysis is to overcome the insufficient power (small sample sizes) of the individual RCTs by statistically pooling the data [15–17]. This effectively increases the number of patients that the data was obtained from, thereby increasing the effective sample size [15]. The major drawback to this pooling is that it is dependent on the quality of RCTs that were included [16]. Meta-analyses are also subject to publication bias. Publication bias refers to the selective publication of research findings based on the magnitude, direction, or statistical significance of research findings [18]. Studies that show small effects or fail to find an effect tend not to get submitted to journals and remain unpublished [18]. Despite these potential limitations, a meta-analysis of high quality RCTs is considered by many to be at the top of the hierarchy of evidence pyramid (see Fig. 2). (See the article by Haines, McKnight, Duku, Perry, and Thoma in this issue.)

Randomized controlled trials

An RCT is an experiment in which individuals are randomly allocated to either receive or not receive an experimental preventative, therapeutic, or diagnostic procedure, and then followed to determine the effect of the intervention on one or more outcomes of interest [19] (Fig. 3). The control group typically receives either an accepted treatment or no treatment at all. The outcomes may be continuous or discrete.

The RCT offers the maximum protection against bias and it is generally regarded as the most scientifically rigorous study design to evaluate the effect of a surgical intervention [20,21]. Historically, surgical

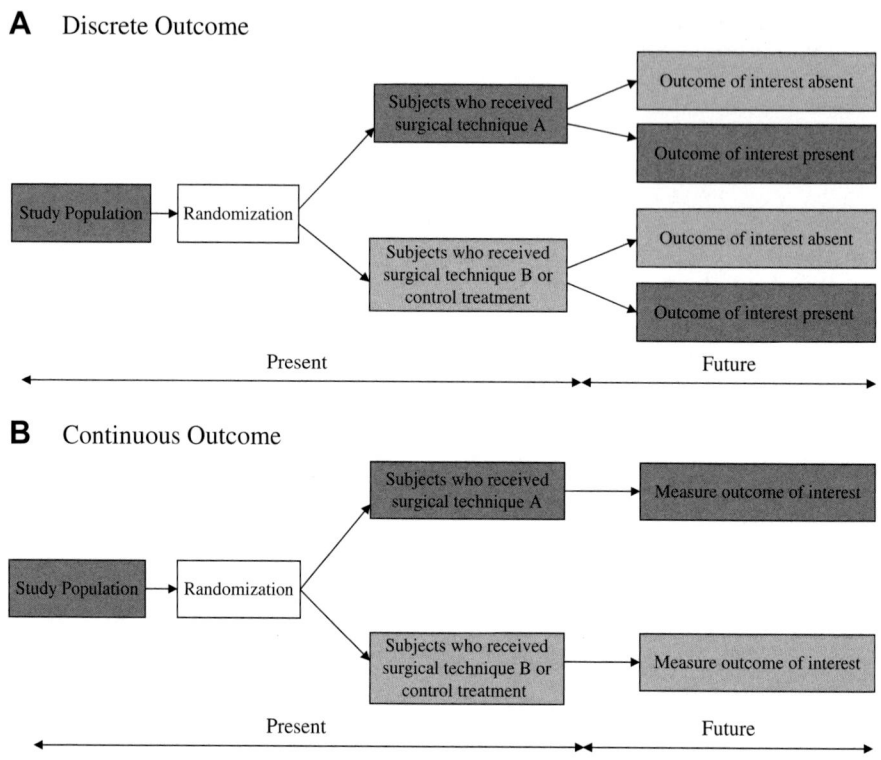

Fig. 3. Randomized controlled trial. (*A*) Discrete outcome. (*B*) Continuous outcome.

RCTs have been performed less often than RCTs comparing medical interventions, partly because using an RCT to evaluate a surgical procedure is difficult and demands special consideration of methodologic issues [22]. Fortunately, RCTs are becoming more common in the surgical literature, as more surgeons are becoming acquainted with the research methodology [22].

Randomization is the only method for balancing both known and unknown prognostic factors between comparison groups [19], and for eliminating selection bias. Although the RCT is the ideal study design to answer questions related to the effects of a novel technique in plastic surgery, as compared with old or prevailing techniques, there are important limitations to consider when evaluating the results of an RCT. (See the article by Thoma, Sprague, Temple, and Archibald in this issue.) Although the randomized study design provides the highest quality evidence, it is also important to consider and understand the strengths and weaknesses of the other study designs (Table 1) [23].

Observational studies: cohort studies and case-controlled studies

An observational study by its very nature observes what happens to individuals during the natural course of events [4]. In contrast to RCTs, in observational studies, the surgeon does not manipulate the study interventions, but rather observes and interprets the outcomes. This section will provide a brief overview of two observational study designs: the cohort study and the case-controlled study. Prospective cohort studies involve the identification and follow-up of individual patients who have received a treatment of interest (Fig. 4) [24]. The investigator selects a group of plastic surgery patients who were treated with Surgery A and compares them to a group of patients who underwent Surgery B. The type of surgery received by each patient is determined by patient and plastic surgeon preference, for various reasons (see Fig. 1). Each patient is followed for a specified time period to determine their outcome (ie, successful or unsuccessful outcomes) and the surgery group with the better outcome or fewer complications is deemed the better treatment option.

A cohort study can also be retrospective or historical if a cohort is identified for whom records of surgical treatment are available and for whom outcomes can be measured after a substantial period of time [25]. In a retrospective cohort study, two or more treatments (techniques) are compared, but the retrospective nature of the data collection and the difficulties involved in comparing

Table 1: Main properties of different study designs

Design	Randomized controlled trials	Cohort studies	Case-controlled studies
Question asked	What are the effects of this intervention?	What are the effects of this intervention?	What were the causes of this event?
Starting point	Intervention status	Intervention status	Event status
Assessment	Event status	Event status	Intervention status
Major strengths	Internal validity: Must have randomization—best way to control bias and confounding; Allows double-blind assessment—best way to control bias.	Feasible when unethical or impossible to randomize. Intervention is assessed before adverse event avoiding bias.	Feasible—can be done with moderate numbers, even on small sample size. Overcomes temporal delays.
Minor weaknesses	Generalizability, feasibility, ethical limitations, long-time scale for some effects.	Threats to internal validity, open to bias, long-time scale for some effects.	Threats to internal validity. Retrospective method limits baseline and intervention information. Exposure may not be recorded.

Data from Elwood M. Critical Appraisal of Epidemiological Studies and Clinical Trials. Second edition. New York: Oxford University Press Inc.; 1998. p. 34.

heterogeneous patient populations limit the believability of the results [1]. For example, consider a hypothetical study in which the investigators performed a retrospective study comparing the outcomes in patients who underwent reconstruction of exposed tibias with free fasciocutaneous flaps versus free muscle flaps. If the investigators found that more patients with free muscle flap reconstructions ended up with below the knee amputations (BKA), does this finding mean that the free muscle flap is inferior to the fasciocutaneous flap? The answer cannot be provided by such a study, as the treating surgeons (and patients) may have chosen one flap or the other for different reasons. The outcome (BKA) may not have been related to the choice of the flap, but rather to the severity of the original trauma or other comorbid conditions.

A case-controlled study, briefly, is a type of observational study that begins with the identification of individuals who already have the outcome of interest (referred to as the cases), and a suitable control group without the outcome event (referred to as the

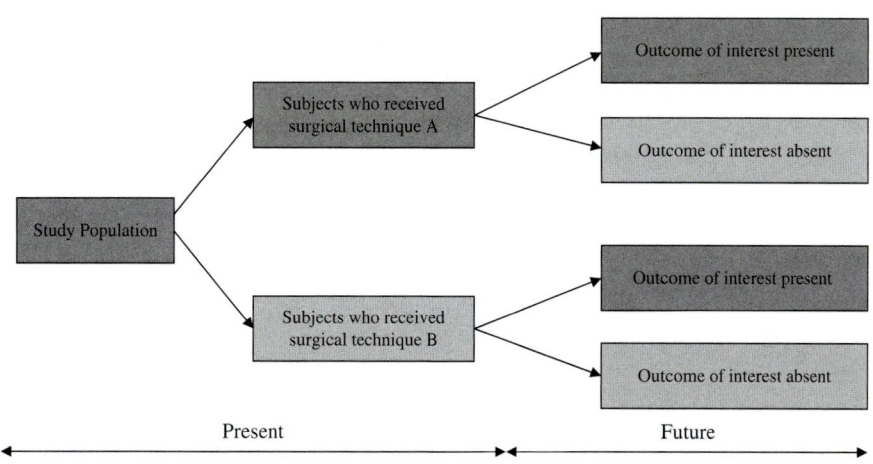

Fig. 4. Cohort study.

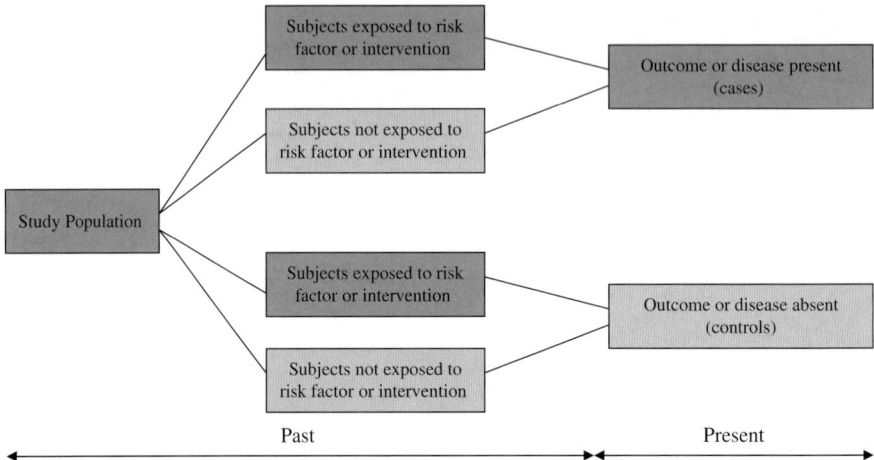

Fig. 5. Case-controlled study.

controls) (Fig. 5) [24]. The investigator then compares the number of individuals with each intervention or prognostic factor of interest in the case group with the corresponding numbers in the control group. Case controlled studies are described as retrospective because they are done looking back in time at information collected about past exposure to possible risk factors. An example of a case-controlled study presently underway at McMaster University is one that addresses the question of whether manual work and single hand injury are risk factors for Dupuytren's disease. The cases are patients with Dupuytren's contracture who are referred to all local plastic surgeons, and the controls are individuals from the same community who are matched with the cases by age and sex. The investigators will collect detailed histories on exposures (manual work and single hand injury) and then compare the exposures rates between the cases and the controls.

Case-controlled studies are not commonly conducted in the surgical literature. They should be used when the outcome under study is rare, when studying outcomes with multiple potential etiologic factors, or looking at outcomes that take a considerable amount of time to develop [26]. Examples of case-controlled studies that have made important contributions in the past include those that established the relationship between thalidomide use in pregnant women and congenital defects in their offspring, asbestos and mesothelioma, and smoking and lung cancer.

The role of observational studies in evaluating competing treatment options is an area of continued debate, as deliberate choice of the treatment for each patient implies that the observed outcome may be caused by differences among patients being given the two different treatments, rather than by the treatment alone [26]. Prospective observational studies overcome some of the limitations of unsystematic clinical observations. However, they are prone to many different biases and limitations. To prevent selection bias, the comparison groups in an observational study should be as similar as possible, except for the factors under study [4].

The positive outcomes frequently achieved from plastic surgical studies, in which surgeons' or patients' choices determined whether or not a patient received the "experimental" surgical treatment versus a "control," may be a result of several causes. The true effect of the experimental treatment is just one of the multiple factors that can account for the outcome. Observational studies often yield misleading results because prognostic factors (age, comorbid conditions, disease, or injury characteristics, for example) usually influence surgeons' recommendations and patients' decisions about submitting themselves to a particular surgical intervention. Previous research has reported that observational studies tend to show larger treatment effects than RCTs, and may show a greater benefit than what actually exists [27–30]. However, some investigators argue that well-constructed observational studies lead to similar conclusions as RCTs [31].

Case reports and series

Unsystematic clinical observations or single case reports represent the lowest level of published clinical evidence. Case reports are uncontrolled, descriptive studies involving a detailed description of an intervention and outcome in one patient [26]. Expansion of the individual case report to include multiple patients with an outcome of interest is referred to as a case series [26]. In a case report or case series involving a technique in plastic surgery, no comparisons are made to a group receiving some other comparator technique. Retrospective case series, unfortunately, are the most common evidence in the plastic surgical literature. By the nature of their design, case reports and case series are limited to making causal inferences about the relationship between risk factors and the outcome of interest [26]. However, case reports and case series can be a valuable stimulus for additional research: they can be hypothesis generating, or may make important observations about a very rare condition [1].

An example of an important case series in the plastic surgical literature is Wei and colleagues [32] work on anterolateral thigh flaps and fibular flaps. In this series, 672 anterolateral thigh flaps were used for head and neck, upper extremity, lower extremity, or trunk reconstruction in 660 patients. This large series demonstrated that the anterolateral thigh flap is a versatile soft-tissue flap in which thickness and volume can be adjusted for the extent of the defect, and that it can replace most soft-tissue free flaps in most clinical situations [32]. However, this study does not definitively demonstrate that this flap is superior to another type of flap, such as the scapular flap. Only a side-by-side comparison in an RCT can address this question.

Basic science or physiologic studies

Basic science or physiologic studies represent low level of evidence for treatment decisions. However, physiologic studies, such as experiments on bone healing, offer valuable insight into how systems may work and are used to generate hypotheses. The early experimental work by Ostrup and Fredrickson [33] led, to a great degree, to the adoption of the free vascularized bone free flaps. This eventually led to the salvaging of mangled lower extremities and later, to the reconstruction of segmental oromandibular defects with vascularized bone grafts. The investigations of the vascular anatomy of the abdomen [34] led, to some degree, to the evolution of various free flaps harvested from the lower abdomen for postmastectomy reconstruction (ie, deep inferior epigastric perforator, superficial inferior epigastric artery, and muscle sparing free flaps) [35–39].

Limitations of using the hierarchy of evidence

Concepts of study methodology are important to consider when placing a study into the levels of evidence [40]. There are some experts who advocate dividing the hierarchy levels into sublevels based in part on study methodology, while others suggest that poor methodology should move a study down a level [41,42]. For instance, one RCT could be considered a very high-level study while another RCT may be considered lower because of methodologic limitations [40]. The rigor with which a study is conducted plays a significant role in how believable the results may be.

Not all case-controlled, cohort, or randomized studies are performed to the same standards and thus, if done multiple times, may have different results, because of both chance and confounding variables and biases [40]. While it is important to look closely at the methods section of a paper to see how the study was conducted, it must be remembered that if something has not been reported as being done (such as the method of randomization), it does not necessarily mean it was not done [43]. This illustrates the importance of tools such as the Consolidated Standards of Reporting Trials (CONSORT) statement for reporting trials, which attempts to improve the quality of reporting [44]. The CONSORT statement was developed by a group of clinical trialists, biostatisticians, epidemiologists, and biomedical editors as a means to improve the quality of reports of RCTs [44].

The hierarchy of evidence implies a clear course of action for plastic surgeons addressing specific research questions. They should strive for the highest available evidence and assess the quality of the study methodology. While data derived from RCTs are considered to be the highest level of evidence, it is important to recognize that not all clinical questions can be answered with an RCT. The popular belief that only the RCT produces trustworthy results, and that all observational studies are misleading, provides a disservice to patient care, clinical investigation, and the education of health care professionals [31]. In many situations, such as in questions of harm causation, an RCT is not feasible, necessary, or appropriate. In plastic surgery, lesser forms of evidence have provided many insights that would not have been possible with RCTs. In addition, observational studies, case series and reports, and basic science studies can generate highly significant hypotheses for future research.

Grading the strength of a body of evidence

In addition to assessing the quality of individual clinical research studies, it is also critical to be able to collectively evaluate an entire body of evidence related to a treatment or technique of interest. Grading the strength of a body of evidence incorporates judgments of study quality, but also includes how confident one is that a finding is true, and whether the same finding has been detected by others using different studies or different people [4]. Thus, grading evidence strength stops at the dashed line in Fig. 6 [4]. Only by incorporating population-specific information, such as regional, racial, and clinical setting differences (akin to generalizability) does one derive a clinical or treatment guideline [4].

The Agency for Health Care Research and Quality recently conducted an extensive review of methods to assess health care research results (Table 2) [4]. The investigators provided a detailed description of the characteristics of seven systems that can be used to grade the strength of a body of research evidence. The National Health Service Center for Evidence Based Medicine's system to grade the strength of the evidence is based on the hierarchy of research design, with some attention to risk and bias [4]. These complex systems' criteria to rate levels of evidence vary by one of the four areas under consideration (therapy, prognosis, diagnosis, and economic analysis).

Systems for rating the strength of a body of evidence are not uniform, and this variability complicates the task of selecting one or more systems for universal use. In addition, approaches for characterizing the strength of the evidence seem to be getting longer and more complex with time, which can make the task of evaluating research difficult and cumbersome. The majority of the grading systems described above are based on the hierarchy of study design, but they also include assessment of the methodologic quality of the research. Reliance on the hierarchy of evidence, without consideration of the methodologic quality, is increasingly seen as unacceptable, and future quality rating systems will call for approaches like those identified above. Selecting among the evidence grading systems will depend on the reason for measuring the strength of the evidence and the type of study being evaluated [4].

Evidence-based plastic surgery

Evidence-based plastic surgery is defined as the integration of the best research evidence with clinical expertise and patient values into clinical decision making. It can also be defined as the conscientious, explicit, and judicious use of current best evidence in making decisions about the care of individual patients. Evidence-based plastic surgery emphasizes the need to properly evaluate the efficacy of plastic surgical interventions before accepting them as standard surgical practice. It involves the process of systematically finding, appraising, and using research findings as the basis for clinical decisions.

There are two fundamental principles of evidence-based plastic surgery. First, the evidence alone is never sufficient to make a clinical decision because plastic surgeons must always trade the benefits and the risks, inconvenience, and costs associated with alternative techniques or procedures, and in doing so also take the patient's values and preferences into consideration. Second, evidence-based plastic surgery requires a hierarchy of evidence to guide clinical decision-making.

The *Users' Guide to the Medical Literature* that appeared in *the Journal of the American Medical Association*, and the recent installments of the *User's Guide to the Surgical Literature* in the *Canadian Journal of Surgery*, provide plastic surgeons with the tools to critically appraise the quality of the plastic surgery research and apply the evidence. Specialized resources, such as summaries of individual studies, systematic reviews, and evidence-based clinical guidelines can help clinicians access the best available evidence [26].

For those who conduct clinical research in plastic surgery, the authors advocate using the study designs at the top of the pyramid (see Fig. 2)—and specifically RCTs with large sample sizes—to achieve narrow confidence intervals. These studies take longer to complete and require greater resources on the short term basis; however, they have the advantage of answering clinically important questions definitively, resulting in saved resources over a long term basis.

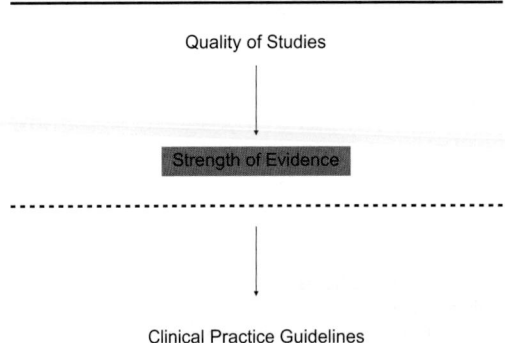

Fig. 6. Continuum from study quality through strength of evidence to guideline. Development. The dashed line is the theoretical dividing line between summarizing the scientific literature and developing a clinical practice guideline. Below the dashed line, guideline developers would decide whether the evidence represents all the relevant subsets of the populations (or settings, or types of clinicians) for whom the guideline is being developed. (*Adapted from* West S, King V, Carey TS, et al. Systems to rate the strength of scientific evidence. Evidence report/technology assessment no. 47. AHRQ Publication No. 02-E016. Rockville, MD: Agency for Healthcare Research and Quality. 2002.)

Table 2: **Grading the evidence**

Author	Grading system
Gyorkos et al, 1994 [45]	Overall assessment of level of evidence based on: • The validity of the individual studies • The strength of association between the intervention and outcomes of interest • Precision of the estimate of strength of association • The variability in finding from independent studies of the same or similar interventions
Clarke & Oxman, 1999 [46]	Questions to consider regarding the strength of inference about the effectiveness of an intervention in the context of a systematic review of clinical trials include: • How good is the quality of the included trials? • How large and significant are the observed effects? • How consistent are the effects across trials? • Is there a clear dose-response relationship? • Is the indirect evidence that supports the inference? • Are there other plausible competing explanations of the observed effects?
Briss et al, 2000 [47]	Evidence of effectiveness is based on: • Execution • Design suitability • Number of studies • Consistency • Effect size
Greer et al, 2000 [48]	Four grades: • Grade I includes evidence from studies of strong design • Grade II includes evidence from studies of strong design, but there is some uncertainty because of inconsistencies or concern about generalizability, bias, research design flaws, or sample size • Grade III has evidence from a limited number of studies of weaker design • Grade IV is the support solely from informed medical competitors based on clinical experience without substantiation from the published literature
Guyatt et al, 2000 [49]	Hierarchy of research design: • N of 1 (single patient) randomized controlled trials • Systematic reviews of RCTs • Single RCTs • Systematic reviews of observational studies addressing patient important-outcomes • Physiologic studies • Unsystematic clinical observations
Harris et al, 2001 [50]	Hierarchy of research design: • I – Evidence from at least one properly conducted RCT • II-1 – Well designed controlled trial without randomization • II-2 – Well designed cohort or case-controlled studies • II-3 – Multiple time series with or without the intervention • III – Opinions of respected authorities based on clinical experience, descriptive studies, and case reports, or reports of expert committees

Summary

Understanding the hierarchy of evidence and study design is a fundamental component of successfully practicing evidence-based plastic surgery. There is an abundance of plastic surgery literature available, and plastic surgeons need to be able to efficiently and effectively evaluate this literature to be able to apply the evidence to the care of individual patients. This article should provide plastic surgeons with a better understanding of the strengths and weaknesses of the various study designs.

References

[1] Urshel J, Goldsmith C, Tandan V, et al. User's guide to evidence-based surgery: how to use an article evaluating surgical interventions. Can J Surg 2001;44:95–100.

[2] Guyatt G, Cairns J, Churchill D, et al. ['Evidence-Based Medicine Working Group']. "Evidence-based medicine. A new approach to teaching the practice of medicine." JAMA 1992;268: 2420–5.

[3] Thoma A, Sprague S. Methodological issues in the comparison of microsurgical flaps/techniques in head and neck reconstruction. Clin Plast Surg 2005;32:347–59.

[4] West S, King V, Carey TS, et al. Systems to Rate the Strength of Scientific Evidence. Evidence Report/Technology Assessment No. 47 (Prepared by the Research Triangle Institute-University of North Carolina Evidence-based Practice Center under Contract No. 290-97-0011). AHRQ Publication No. 02-E016. Rockville, MD: Agency for Healthcare Research and Quality; April 2002.

[5] Canadian Task Force on the Periodic Health Examination. Can Med Assoc J 1979;121: 1193–254.

[6] Sacket DL. Rules of evidence and clinical recommendations on the use of antithrombotic agents. Chest 1986;89(2 Suppl):2S–3S.

[7] Woolfe K. Using information to optimize case management. AAOHN J 1990;38:504–6.

[8] Cook DJ, Guyatt GH, Laupacis A, et al. Rules of evidence and clinical recommendations on the use of antithrombotic agents. Chest 1992;102:305S–11S.

[9] Guyatt GH, Sackett DL, Sinclair JC, et al. Users' Guides to the Medical Literature. IX. A method for grading health care recommendations. Evidence-Based Medicine Working Group. JAMA 1995;274:1800–4.

[10] Cochrane A. Effectiveness and efficiency: random reflections on health services. Nuffield Provincial Hospitals Trust. London; 1972.

[11] Oxman AD, Guyatt GH. Guidelines for reading literature reviews. Can Med Assoc J 1988;138: 697–703.

[12] Oxman AD, Sackett DL, Guyatt GH. Users' Guides to the Medical Literature. I. How to get started. The Evidence-Based Medicine Working Group. JAMA 1993;270:2093–5.

[13] Meakins JL. Evidence-based clinical practice. Can J Surg 2000;43:404–5.

[14] Cook DJ, Mulrow CD, Haynes RB. Systematic reviews: synthesis of best evidence for clinical decisions. Ann Intern Med 1997;126:376–80.

[15] Fleiss JL. The statistical basis of meta-analysis. Stat Methods Med Res 1993;2:121–45.

[16] Sackett DL, Haynes RB, Guyatt GH, et al. Clinical epidemiology: a basic science for clinical medicine. Boston: Little, Brown and Company; 1991.

[17] Sackett DL, Richardson WS, Rosenberg WM, et al. Evidence based medicine: how to practice and teach EBM. New York: Churchill Livingstone; 1997.

[18] Montori VM, Smieja M, Guyatt GH. Publication bias: a brief review for clinicians. Mayo Clin Proc 2000;75:1284–8.

[19] American Medical Association. Users' Guides to the medical literature: a manual for evidence-based practice. In: Guyatt GH, Rennie D, editors. 2nd edition. Chicago: American Medical Association Press; 2001. p. 55–79, 686.

[20] Coditz GA, Miller JN, Mosteller F. How study design affects outcomes in comparisons of therapy. [I. Medical. and II. Surgical]. Stat Med 1989;8: 411–66.

[21] Schultz KF, Chalmers I, Hayes RJ, et al. Empirical evidence of bias: dimensions of methodological quality associated with estimates of treatment effects in controlled trials. JAMA 1995;273: 408–12.

[22] Thoma A, Farrokhyar F, Bhandari M, et al. [Evidence-Based Surgery Working Group]. Users' Guide to the Surgical Literature: how to assess a randomized controlled study. Can J Surg 2004;47:200–8.

[23] Elwood M. Critical appraisal of epidemiological studies and clinical trials. 2nd edition. New York: Oxford University Press Inc.; 1998.

[24] Streiner DL, Norman GR. PDQ Epidemiology. St. Louis (MO): Mosby—Yearbook Inc.; 1997.

[25] Gordis L. Epidemiology. Philadelphia: W.B. Saunders Company; 1996.

[26] Brighton B, Bhandari M, Tornetta P, et al. Hierarchy of evidence: from case reports to randomized controlled trials. Clin Orthop Relat Res 2003;413:19–24.

[27] Sacks HS, Chalmers TC, Smith H Jr. Sensitivity and specificity of clinical trials: randomized v historical controls. Arch Intern Med 1983;143: 753–5.

[28] Chalmers TC, Celano P, Sacks HS, et al. Bias in treatment assignment in controlled clinical trials. N Engl J Med 1983;309:1358–61.

[29] Colditz GA, Miller JN, Mosteller F. How study design affects outcomes in comparisons of therapy. I: Medical. Stat Med 1989;8:441–54.

[30] Emerson JD, Burdick E, Hoaglin DC, et al. An empirical study of the possible relation of treatment differences to quality scores in controlled randomized clinical trials. Control Clin Trials 1990;11:339–52.

[31] Concato J, Shah N, Howitz RI. Randomized controlled trials, observational studies, and hierarchy of research designs. N Engl J Med 2000; 342:1887–92.

[32] Wei FC, Jain V, Celik N, et al. Have we found an ideal soft-tissue flap? An experience with 672 anterolateral thigh flaps. Plast Reconstr Surg 2002; 109:2219–26.

[33] Ostrup LT, Fredrickson JM. Distant transfer of a free living bone graft by microvascular anastomoses. Plast Reconstr Surg 1974;54:274–85.

[34] Boyd JB, Taylor GI, Corlett R. The vascular territories of the superior epigastric and the deep inferior epigastric systems. Plast Reconstr Surg 1984;73:1–16.

[35] Chevray PM. Breast reconstruction with superficial inferior epigastric artery flaps: a prospective comparison with TRAM and DIEP flaps. Plast Reconstr Surg 2004;114:1077–83.

[36] Cheng MH, Lin JY, Ulusal BG, et al. Comparisons of resource costs and success rates between immediate and delayed breast reconstruction using DIEP or SIEA flaps under a well-controlled clinical trial. Plast Reconstr Surg 2006;117:2139–42.

[37] Vermeulen P, Fabre G, Vandevoort M. The superficial inferior epigastric artery flap for breast reconstruction. Results and complications in 43 cases. Presented at the American Society for Reconstructive Microsurgery meeting. Fajardo, Puerto Rico. January 15–18, 2005.

[38] Craigie JE, Allen RJ, Heitland AS. Autogenous breast reconstruction with the superficial inferior epigastric artery flap. American Society for Reconstructive Microsurgery meeting. Kawai, Hawaii. January 11–14, 2003.

[39] Vega SJ, Bossert RP, Serletti JM. Improving outcomes in bilateral breast reconstruction using autogenous tissue. Ann Plast Surg 2006;56:487–90.

[40] Bhandari M, Petrisor B. The hierarchy of evidence: levels and grades of recommendation. Indian Journal of Orthopaedics 2007;41:11–5.

[41] Atkins D, Best D, Briss PA, et al. Grading quality of evidence and strength of recommendations. BMJ 2004;328:1490.

[42] Phillips B, Ball C, Sackett DL, et al. Levels of evidence and grades of recommendation. Centre for evidence-based medicine: Oxford-centre for evidence based medicine. GENERIC; 1998.

[43] Devereaux PJ, Manns BJ, Ghali WA, et al. The reporting of methodological factors in randomized controlled trials and the association with a journal policy to promote adherence to the Consolidated Standards of Reporting Trials (CONSORT) checklist. Control Clin Trials 2002;23:380–8.

[44] Moher D, Schulz KF, Altman DG, [CONSORT Group]. The CONSORT statement: revised recommendations for improving the quality of reports of parallel group randomised trials. JAMA 2001;285:1987–91.

[45] Gyorkos TW, Tannenbaum TN, Abrahamowicz M, et al. An approach to the development of practice guidelines for community health interventions. Can J Public Health. Revue Canadienne De Sante Publique 1994;85(Suppl 1):S8–13.

[46] Clarke M, Oxman AD. Cochrane Reviewer's Handbook 4.0. The Cochrane Collaboration; 1999.

[47] Briss PA, Zaza S, Pappaioanou M, et al. Developing an evidence-based Guide to Community Preventive Services—methods. The Task Force on Community Preventive Services. Am J Prev Med 2000;18:35–43.

[48] Greer N, Mosser G, Logan G, et al. A practical approach to evidence grading. Jt Comm J Qual Improv 2000;26:700–12.

[49] Guyatt GH, Haynes RB, Jaeschke RZ, et al. Users' Guides to the Medical Literature: XXV. Evidence-based medicine: principles for applying the Users' Guides to patient care. Evidence-Based Medicine Working Group. JAMA 2000;284:1290–6.

[50] Harris RP, Helfand M, Woolf SH, et al. Current methods of the U.S. Preventive Services Task Force: a review of the process. Am J Prev Med 2001;20:21–35.

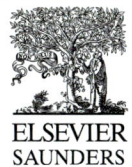

The Role of Systematic Reviews in Clinical Research and Practice

Ted Haines, MD, MSc, FRCPC[a], Leslie McKnight, MSc[b],
Eric Duku, MSc, PStat[c], Lenora Perry, BSc[a,d],
Achilleas Thoma, MD, MSc, FRCS(C), FACS[a,b,e],*

- Types of reviews
- Steps in conducting a systematic review
  The research question
  The research protocol
  The literature search
  Screening and evaluation of study quality

  Data extraction
  Data analysis
  Results and interpretation
- Summary
- References

Physicians need to be informed about the effectiveness of the treatments and accuracy of the tests that they use, as part of the practice of evidence-based medicine. Increasingly, patients are explicitly seeking this information. They commonly come to their referral appointment with a few abstracts, or with questions about a major study they have heard about. For the surgeon, applying evidence-based medicine means that clinical decision-making is informed by three factors: the interests and preferences of the patient; his or her clinical judgment, experience and skill; and the best available research evidence on the clinical question [1]. This article addresses the third of these factors.

The constant demand to keep up with the literature in surgery is becoming a formidable challenge. Not only is it necessary to find time to read the literature, it is important to evaluate what one reads to decide whether it is meaningful to one's practice, and credible enough to incorporate into clinical decision-making [2].

More and more, busy surgeons are relying on systematic reviews to help them keep up with the literature [2]. In a well done systematic review, the findings of all high quality studies pertaining to a particular clinical question are evaluated together to provide more valid information than any one study can. A good systematic review offers the

---

[a] Department of Clinical Epidemiology and Biostatistics, McMaster University, Hamilton Health Sciences Centre, 1200 Main Street West, Hamilton, ON L8N 3Z5, Canada
[b] Department of Surgery, Division of Plastic Surgery, St. Joseph's Healthcare, 50 Charlton Avenue East, Hamilton, ON L8N 4A6, Canada
[c] Department of Psychiatry and Behavioural Neurosciences, Offord Centre for Child Studies, McMaster University, Chedoke Division, Patterson Building Room 217, 1200 Main Street West, Hamilton, ON L8N 3Z5, Canada
[d] Department of Medicine, University of Western Ontario, London Health Sciences Centre, 339 Windermere Road, London, ON L8P 3A9, Canada
[e] Surgical Outcomes Research Centre (SOURCE), McMaster University, St. Joseph's Healthcare, 50 Charlton Avenue East, Hamilton, ON L8N 4A6, Canada
* Corresponding author. 206 James Street South, Suite 101, Hamilton, ON L8P 3A9, Canada
E-mail address: athoma@mcmaster.ca (A. Thoma).

"users" of clinical research the best available evidence to use in their clinical practice. For the "doers" of surgical research, it summarizes the evidence, which may spark a new research project to answer any questions that remain unanswered by the systematic review.

Types of reviews

At the Potsdam Conference in 1995, methodologic guidelines for systematic reviews were determined. In those guidelines, systematic reviews are defined as "the application of scientific strategies that limit bias to the systematic assembly, critical appraisal, and synthesis of all relevant studies on a specific topic" [1]. Systematic reviews are performed to produce an unbiased overview of the literature. Accordingly, they can be used to inform evidence-based decisions [3,4]. As discussed below, they are distinguished from nonsystematic narrative reviews by a detailed methods section that should provide enough information for the study to be reproduced [3].

It is important to recognize that systematic reviews are different from "narrative" reviews or "expert opinion" articles and editorials (Table 1). In these types of reviews, sometimes written by invitation and often by authoritative individuals, an overview of a topic is given in its broad context, with insights based on personal perspective. These types of articles can be informative and helpful [3,5–7]; however, narrative reviews and expert opinion reports do not involve a systematic method of selection and evaluation of the literature.

Not only can systematic reviews of original research facilitate clinical decision-making, but also systematic reviews of review articles themselves can be helpful in addressing a large body of conflicting literature. For example, there is ongoing controversy about the comparative effectiveness of open carpal tunnel release (OCTR) and endoscopic carpal tunnel release (ECTR) in treating carpal tunnel syndrome [8]. Thoma and colleagues [8] conducted a systematic review of review articles to determine if reviews of high methodologic quality have been published on the relative effectiveness of ECTR and OCTR and to abstract and summarize their findings. The methodology for conducting systematic reviews of reviews is analogous to that of systematic reviews. The main difference is in the assessment of the methodologic quality of articles. Assessing the quality of systematic or narrative reviews should be performed using a validated quality assessment scale designed specifically for review articles, such as the Oxman and Guyatt index [9] or the scale of Hoving and colleagues [10]. These types of scales assess the rigor of the methods for searching of the literature, selection and methodologic appraisal of articles, and data abstraction and synthesis of results.

In a meta-analysis, the results of the primary studies that meet the standards for inclusion in a review are mathematically pooled to give a result that is more precise because of the overall increase in numbers of study participants contributing data. For example, none of several small studies conducted to compare ECTR to OCTR were able to resolve controversy over which technique leads to better results. Answers emerged once the results from all studies were pooled in a meta-analysis [11].

Systematic reviews and meta-analyses of the effectiveness of treatments can be performed based on randomized controlled trials (RCTs) or observational studies [3,12,13]. However, RCTs are the traditional study design of choice for primary studies used in meta-analyses, as they are the most likely to be valid [6,14,15]. Procedures, such as blinding and concealment of treatment allocation, minimize the potential for systematic error (see the article by Thoma, Sprague, Temple, and Archibald in this issue). However, in recent years progress has been made in improving the quality of observational studies and developing statistical methods for performing

Table 1: Differences between narrative and systematic reviews

Narrative review	Systematic review
Research question is often broad	Well-focused clinical question
Search strategy is not defined or systematic	Explicit search strategy, outlining study inclusion or exclusion criteria
Article selection is not systematic	Article selection is specific to inclusion or exclusion criteria
Appraisal of study quality may not be performed	Articles are critically appraised and strengths and weaknesses documented
Qualitative summary of findings	Qualitative or quantitative analysis of findings

Adapted from Cook DJ, Mulrow CD, Haynes RB. Systematic reviews: synthesis of best evidence for clinical practice decisions. Ann Intern Med 1997;126:376-80; with permission.

meta-analyses on results of observational studies [6,15,16].

Frequently, it is not feasible to conduct a meta-analysis. If the data accumulated from the primary studies are of poor quality or too heterogeneous to be reasonably pooled, a quantitative meta-analysis needs to be abandoned in favor of a qualitative systematic review [1,6,13,17]. The term "heterogeneity" refers to differences in study populations and methods. For example, it may be inappropriate to pool data from a population of children with that from an adult population, depending on the research question. Furthermore, the methodologic quality of RCTs varies. In a systematic review by Martou and colleagues [18] of studies on surgical techniques used to treat osteoarthritis of the carpometacarpal joint of the thumb, meta-analysis was not possible because of the poor quality and heterogeneity among the primary studies, most of which were observational. In instances such as these, one important benefit of the systematic review is that it draws attention to the need for well-conducted RCTs on the topic.

Not all research designs are equal in their ability to generate convincing evidence. A well-conducted systematic review or meta-analysis provides the highest level of evidence to support an answer to a clinical question (see the article by Sprague, McKay, and Thoma in this issue). When the results of the individual studies are valid, a meta-analysis is a powerful procedure that gives an end result that is more precise than any one study alone. The increased power of the meta-analysis lies in the pooling of data from smaller studies to increase the overall numbers of subjects. The result of a meta-analysis can help resolve controversy over whether a true effect exists, when results have been variable in single studies, or can validate a statistically non-significant but clinically important result in a small study [6,13,15].

Steps in conducting a systematic review

It is important to be aware that to carry out a systematic review well is a labor intensive and time-consuming endeavor [12,15]. A helpful approach is to break it down into a step-by-step process (Table 2), with the first step being the formulation of the research question.

The research question

Although it may seem an over-statement, the formatting and focus of the question the review is intended to answer is critical. Clarifying the study question at the very beginning of the process will guide the development of the protocol for the systematic review. A properly constructed question about treatment will describe: (1) the patient population you are targeting, (2) the nature of the intervention, (3) what the comparative intervention is (this may be a different treatment, or may be no treatment, a placebo, or a historical comparator), (4) the outcome of interest, and (5) the time horizon (time required to measure the desired outcome) (see the article by Thoma, McKnight, McKay, and Haines in this issue). Outcomes are usually the occurrence or prevention of an event, but may include such important issues as cost-effectiveness or patient satisfaction [18,19].

The decision about which study designs to include in the review will depend on the nature and intention of the review. Systematic reviews aim to: (a) summarize the existing literature; (b) resolve conflicts or controversies in the literature; (c) clarify the results of multiple studies; or (d) evaluate the need for further studies.

Because there may be few RCTs available on a topic in surgery, it may be decided to include all study designs that use a comparative group [3,12,13,15]; however, there are disadvantages to this decision. There is an increased risk of bias in observational studies, even when adjustments have been made in the primary studies for known confounders that will impact the results. In addition, the inclusion of observational studies may make an overall meta-analysis impossible because of heterogeneity in methods [20]. Alternatively, the decision may be to include only RCTs in the review.

The inclusion and exclusion criteria usually include study characteristics, population characteristics, and sometimes aspects such as time period, location, or language [10,13]. Surgical reviews present considerations for inclusion and exclusion criteria that are not encountered in reviews of the effectiveness of medications, such as changes in technology of surgical procedures over time, and the experience or technique of surgeons performing procedures [3,13].

The degree of heterogeneity among studies will be influenced by the strictness of the inclusion and exclusion criteria that are established for the review. Establishing broad inclusion criteria can increase the number of studies selected for analysis, and may increase the generalized nature of results because fewer study populations or study procedures are ruled out of the analysis. However, the cost of the increased generalized nature is increased heterogeneity, such that pooling results may not be feasible because of important variations in study characteristics [3,12].

The research protocol

The research question should act as a reference point and guide the development of a research

Table 2: **Step-by-step guide to performing a systematic review of the literature**

Steps	Key considerations
Step 1. Forming the research question	A clear, concise research question should be formed using the acronym PICOT (Population, Intervention, Comparative, Outcomes, Time Horizon). This question will underlie the methods of the research protocol.
Step 2. The research protocol	The protocol detailing the literature search strategy, study screening, selection and evaluation, and data extraction and analysis must be defined before study initiation.
Step 3. Literature search	Databases, search terms and inclusion and exclusion criteria must be decided upon before the search is initiated. The research question will determine what types of studies will be included in the search.
Step 4. Screening and evaluation of study quality	Two independent assessors should perform study screening and selection, and evaluation of study quality. Reasons for study exclusion must be documented.
Step 5. Data extraction	The data extracted from articles will depend on the research question you are trying to answer. Data extraction forms should be used to facilitate data collection.
Step 6. Data analysis	Random-effects model is the most realistic statistical model for meta-analysis in surgical research. If meta-analysis is not feasible, the investigators do qualitative analysis consensually. A statistician familiar with clinical aspects of the review should be involved in the study from the beginning stages.
Step 7. Review and interpretation of results	Guidelines such as Quality of Reports of Meta-analysis (QUORUM) can be used for reporting results. The strengths and weaknesses of included studies should be discussed, as well as the strengths and weaknesses (potential biases) of the current review.

protocol. The protocol outlines what types of studies will best address the question and meet the requirements for the review, what inclusion and exclusion criteria will be used in the final selection of included articles, and what outcomes to focus on. In the protocol, the details of methods are defined for the literature search, study screening and selection, quality evaluation, data extraction, and synthesis and interpretation. The establishment of these methods clearly at the outset in a study protocol is critical to prevent biases from entering the review process [3,6,12,13,15].

The literature search

The literature search must be as exhaustive as possible, seeking out primary studies and previously completed reviews on the topic in both published and unpublished literature. It is important to be aware of potential sources of bias that can evolve from a hastily or carelessly performed literature search.

Publication bias is a well-known problem affecting systematic reviews. Studies with statistically significant results are often more likely to end up being published, while studies with inconclusive or negative findings are more likely to be found in the "gray" literature [3,12,20]. Gray literature includes such works as theses, conference proceedings, company reports, and studies published in less prominent, hard-to-find journals [12,20]. Research by McAuley and colleagues [21] reports that failure to include gray literature in a search may lead to exaggeration of effect size in the meta-analysis by an average of 12%. This exaggeration can be compounded by the practice of including studies in the review that are found by searching the bibliographies of published studies, as these are more likely to support the findings of the original study [15].

Publication bias will become less problematic over time as journal editors are now avoiding the use of statistical significance as a criterion for publication [12]. In addition, prospective registry in a recognized searchable and publicly available database, such as clinicaltrials.gov, is now a requirement for publication for many journals for studies that have a comparison group [4].

Funnel plots and other statistical tests are now commonly used in meta-analyses to detect whether publication bias has had an impact on the results [3,13,20]. The funnel plot is based on research that has shown that large studies are most likely to be published and published quickly, while smaller studies may be published only if they have significant results [22]. Egger and colleagues [23] developed a statistical test to detect publication bias based on the use of a scatter plot (that takes the shape of a funnel) of effect estimates of studies. The scatter plot highlights differences between large and small studies.

Another source of bias to watch for comes from the inclusion of duplicate studies resulting from multiple publications of the same or overlapping studies. Duplications can be eliminated at this stage based on predetermined criteria, or highlighted for elimination by reviewers at a later stage, but only one publication—generally, the most recent—from duplicated studies should be used in the systematic review [10,20,24]. Limiting a search to English language studies may also lead to bias, because positive studies are more likely to be published in English [12,23]. While the identification of non-English studies brings added effort with respect to translation, it is becoming less and less acceptable to base a systematic review on only English language studies [2]. For example, a recent meta-analysis of RCTs that compared OCTR to ECTR used data after translating into English some of the original studies, which were published in French, German, Dutch, and Portuguese [11].

In performing a review, time and resources available may determine the extent and exhaustiveness of the literature search. In writing up the review, it is important to include the details of the literature search so that readers may judge its quality. Although searching the literature for potentially relevant articles is a time-consuming part of the review [3,25], a well-defined question will make the literature search more efficient. The wording of the question will provide targeted keywords to use in your search [14,26].

The search must use at the very least two, and preferably numerous, bibliographic databases. The largest and most readily accessible database is the National Library of Medicine's freely available MEDLINE, offered on the World Wide Web through PubMed, or through institutional interfaces (for a fee), such as OVID, SilverPlatter, and others. MEDLINE's PubMed interface has many convenient features that are constantly being updated and improved, and the ever-enlarging database offers upwards of 10,000,000 citations. However, the use of MEDLINE only tends to restrict the search to primarily English language studies with a North American focus. Embase is a European database that will capture studies in other languages, but places its emphasis on treatment and pharmacology, so it may be less useful for retrieving studies in surgery [12,19]. One of the best resources for high quality RCTs in all languages, as well as ongoing and unpublished studies, is the Cochrane Central Register of Controlled Trials, part of the Cochrane Library [12]. A librarian can direct you to other databases available at your institution, suitable to your particular literature search that will cover the pertinent biomedical references that may not be contained in any of the above resources.

A high level of expertise is required to understand the technical aspects of data structure and databases, to narrow the search to manageable numbers without losing relevant citations, to access the gray literature, to manage the references, and to document retrieval methods for the eventual write-up of the review. It is advisable to have a professional medical librarian or information specialist set up the search terms, using the key words you have identified, and conduct the search [2,27].

Screening and evaluation of study quality

The literature search will often result in a large number of citations. Many of these can be discarded by reading the title and abstract using broad screening criteria, leaving a group of titles and abstracts of uncertain or potential relevance. Ideally, two reviewers conduct this process of study identification, but project resources may not permit this. For the studies identified as potentially relevant, full articles are retrieved. These need to be evaluated by at least two reviewers, using predetermined inclusion and exclusion criteria as discussed above, as well as methods to arrive at consensus, in case of disagreement, to decide which ones will be included in the review [21]. Once studies are selected for inclusion, they should be assessed for quality by at least two investigators working independently [3,10,15,28,29]. Generally, selected articles will vary greatly in quality.

Quality assessments of the methodology of individual selected studies are based on the extent to which bias is minimized. Characteristics to consider are the following: (1) method of group allocation and its concealment, (2) indication of unequal additional treatment or intervention, (3) attention to blinding, (4) objective criteria for assessment of important outcomes, and (4) use of the intention-to-treat principle, whereby all patients must be analyzed in their originally assigned group, regardless of in which group they will ultimately be placed [1].

Attempts have been made to find ways to give more credit or weight to better studies, through the use of scales (eg, the Jadad scale for RCTs, and the Newcastle-Ottawa scale for observational studies) [30–32] and checklists (eg, the Consolidated Standards of Reporting Trials checklist for RCTs and the Strengthening of Reporting of Observational Studies in Epidemiology group checklist for observational studies) [6]. These are helpful tools; however, caution in using them is warranted, as research has shown that the scores can be misleading and reliance on them can alter the results of a meta-analysis [30,33].

The Meta-analysis of Observational Studies in Epidemiology (MOOSE) group suggests the use of sensitivity or subgroup analysis, rather than weighting studies according to a quality score [15,16]. Using this technique, studies are grouped according to levels of quality or clinical characteristics that are thought to possibly influence results. When the groups are analyzed, the results are compared to determine whether or not there are significant differences [3,15,16]. In this way, it can be determined whether or how much a particular study characteristic or design weakness will influence the overall results of a meta-analysis.

It is essential to record the details of the selection process and the reasons for excluding studies, and all stages of the quality assessment, to be completely transparent to future readers of the review [1,15,21].

Data extraction

Data extraction is the tabulation of results from each of the selected studies in a specific format, usually called the "data extraction" form. The form, with details about what information will be extracted from the studies, should be designed as part of the study protocol [15]. The data extraction step may be incorporated into the study selection process, depending on individual study characteristics and preferences of investigators.

Two independent reviewers should perform data extraction. If key data are missing from an article, the authors of the primary study should be contacted. If it is not possible to obtain complete data from the authors, or too much data are missing, the study may need to be withdrawn from the review, with an explanation written into the study records [12].

While data extraction forms will vary according to the research question, common to all forms for a review of treatment effectiveness will be the study title, design, populations, interventions, outcomes, and additional information about the methods, such as length of follow-up [12,15,28]. The major challenge in this step is to get all data into a standardized format so that comparison and pooling of data can be done [15].

Data analysis

Simply stated, a meta-analysis calculates a weighted average of the study effect that is pooled from a group of selected studies. Larger studies have more influence over the summary estimate than smaller ones [15,20].

Two statistical models are commonly used to analyze data for meta-analyses. The fixed-effects model considers only within-study variation, on the assumption that there is a true effect that in theory would be the same for every study, if it were infinitely large. The random-effects model assumes between-study variation exists, as well as within-study variation, such that the true effect estimate for each study will vary. The random-effects model is more realistic, and should be used particularly in surgical research where heterogeneity is likely a result of characteristics unique to surgery, such as variation in surgical technique in a procedure [1,6].

The potential for heterogeneity among studies in a review will be reflected in the range of the results of the selected studies. A wide range may be caused by chance alone, or may be a result of clinical and methodologic differences among studies [3,12,13,20] even though they are measuring the same outcome. Unfortunately, when there are few studies, such as is often the case in surgery reviews, tests for heterogeneity may not have enough power, meaning that they may not be able to identify whether or not there is heterogeneity [15]. For this reason, clinical judgment must play an important role in determining whether a meta-analysis can reasonably be performed, or whether a qualitative, narrative synthesis is more advisable [3,12,13,20].

In a qualitative analysis, judgments on effectiveness are made consensually by the investigators on the basis of articles, which to that point have been rigorously searched, selected, evaluated, and abstracted. Taken into consideration are factors such as sample size, methodologic quality scores, and differences in study methods, outcomes, and durations of follow-up.

A detailed description of statistical procedures and statistical software used for meta-analysis is beyond the scope of this article [34]. A statistician who is also familiar with the clinical aspects of the review should be involved from the beginning of the study.

Results and interpretation

At this stage, the results of the review can be summarized and documented in preparation for publication. Guidelines for reporting results of meta-analyses for both RCTs (QUORUM) and for observational studies (MOOSE) should be consulted [16,35]. The methodologic strengths and weaknesses of included studies should be discussed, as well as the merits and limitations of the current systematic review itself. Any clinical recommendations based on the findings of the review should be practical and explicit [1]. Effect sizes and potential impact on practice should be discussed. All stages of the review should be transparently described, so that readers can evaluate its quality [1,15].

Summary

Well-conducted systematic reviews and meta-analyses provide the best quality evidence for clinical decision-making. There are seven critical steps in performing a systematic review:

1. Forming a clear, clinically relevant research question
2. Developing a detailed research protocol
3. Performing an exhaustive systematic search of the available literature
4. Critically appraising the quality of selected articles
5. Extracting relevant data
6. Performing a statistical or qualitative analysis of the extracted results
7. Interpreting the findings, and addressing the strengths and weaknesses of selected articles and of the review itself

References

[1] Cook DJ, Sackett DL, Spitzer WO. Methodologic guidelines for systematic reviews of randomized control trials in health care from the Potsdam Consultation on Meta-Analysis. J Clin Epidemiol 1995;48(1):167–71.
[2] Burton M, Clark M. Systematic reviews of surgical interventions. Surg Clin North Am 2006;86: 101–14.
[3] Sauerland S, Seiler CM. The role of systematic reviews and meta-analysis in evidence based medicine. World J Surg 2005;29:582–7.
[4] Farquhar C, Vail A. Pitfalls in systematic reviews. Curr Opin Obstet Gynecol 2006;18:433–9.
[5] Slavin RE. Best evidence synthesis: an intelligent alternative to meta-analysis. J Clin Epidemiol 1995;48(1):9–18.
[6] Mahid SS, Hornung CA, Minor KS, et al. Systematic reviews and meta-analysis for the surgical scientist. Br J Surg 2006;93:1315–24.
[7] Doig CJ, Rocker G. Retrieving organs from non-heart-beating organ donors: a review of medical and ethical issues. Can J Anaesth 2003;50:1069–76.
[8] Thoma A, Veltri K, Haines T, et al. A systematic review of reviews comparing endoscopic and open carpal tunnel decompression. Plast Reconstr Surg 2004;13:1184–91.
[9] Oxman AD, Guaytt GH. Validation of an index of the quality of review articles. J Clin Epidemiol 1991;44(11):1271–8.
[10] Hoving JL, Gross AR, Gasner D, et al. A critical appraisal of review articles on the effectiveness and conservation treatment of for neck pain. Spine 2001;26:196–205.
[11] Thoma A, Veltri K, Haines T, et al. A meta-analysis of RCTs comparing endoscopic and open CT decompression. Plast Reconstr Surg 2004;114: 1137–46.
[12] Wright RW, Brand RA, Dunn W, et al. How to write a systematic review. Clin Orthop Relat Res 2007;455:23–9.
[13] Ng TT, McGory ML, Ko CL, et al. Meta-analysis in surgery. Arch Surg 2006;141:1125–30.
[14] Thoma A, Sprague S. Methodologic issues in the comparison of microsurgical flaps/techniques in head and neck reconstruction. Clin Plast Surg 2005;32:347–59.
[15] Chung K, Burns PB, Kim M. A practical guide to meta-analysis. J Hand Surg [Am] 2006;31:1671–8.
[16] Stroup DF, Berlin JA, Morton SC, et al. Meta-analysis of observational studies in epidemiology: a proposal for reporting. Meta-analysis Of Observational Studies in Epidemiology (MOOSE) group. JAMA 2000;283:2008–12.
[17] Gerritsen AA, de Vet HC, Scholten RJ, et al. Enabling meta-analysis in systematic reviews on carpal tunnel syndrome. J Hand Surg [Am] 2002;27:828–32.
[18] Martou G, Veltri K, Thoma A. Surgical treatment of osteoarthritis of the carpometacarpal joint of the thumb: a systematic review. Plast Reconstr Surg 2004;114:421–32.
[19] McCulloch P, Badenoch D. Finding and appraising evidence. Surg Clin North Am 2006;86: 41–57.
[20] Khoshdel A, Attia J, Carney SL. Basic concepts in meta-analysis: a primer for clinicians. Int J Clin Pract 2006;60:1287–94.
[21] McAuley L, Pham B, Tugwell P, et al. Does the inclusion of grey literature influence estimates of intervention effectiveness reported in meta-analyses? Lancet 2000;356:1228–31.
[22] Egger M, Schneider M, Davey Smith G. Spurious precision? Meta-analysis of observational studies. BMJ 1998;316:140–4.
[23] Egger M, Davey Smith G, Schneider M, et al. Bias in meta-analysis detected by a simple, graphical test. BMJ 1997;315:629–34.
[24] Johnson SH. 2002 Duplicate publication, Part 2: a case analysis. Nurse Author Ed 2002;12(4):7–8.
[25] Allen IE, Olkin I. Estimating time to conduct a meta-analysis from number of citations retrieved. JAMA 1999;282:634–5.
[26] Sackett D, Straus S, Richardson W, et al. Evidence-based medicine: how to practice and teach EBM. Philadelphia: Churchill Livingston; 2000.

[27] McGowan J, Sampson M. Systematic reviews need systematic searchers. J Med Libr Assoc 2005;93:74–80.

[28] Berman NG, Parker RA. Meta-analysis: neither quick nor easy. BMC Med Res Methodol 2002;2:10.

[29] Egger M, Smith GD, Phillips AN. Meta-analysis: principles and procedures. BMJ 1997;315: 1533–7.

[30] Moher D, Jadad AR, Nichol G, et al. Assessing the quality of randomized controlled trials: an annotated bibliography of scales and checklists. Control Clin Trials 1995;16:62–73.

[31] Jadad AR, Moore RA, Carroll D, et al. Assessing the quality of reports of randomized clinical trials: is blinding necessary? Control Clin Trials 1996;17:1–12.

[32] Wells GA, Shea B, O'Connell D, et al. The Newcastle-Ottawa scale (NOS) for assessing the quality of nonrandomised studies in meta-analyses. In: Proceedings of the Third Symposium on Systematic Reviews: beyond the basics. UK: Oxford; July 2000.

[33] Juni P, Witschi A, Bloch R, et al. The hazards of scoring the quality of clinical trials for meta-analysis. JAMA 1999;282:1054–60.

[34] Fleiss JL. The statistical basis of meta-analysis. Stat Methods Med Res 1993;2:121–45.

[35] Moher D, Cook DJ, Eastwood S, et al. Improving the quality of reports of meta-analyses of randomised controlled trials: the QUOROM statement. Quality of Reporting of Meta-analyses. Lancet 1999;354:1896–900.

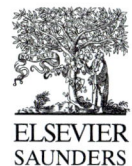

Clinical Research in Breast Surgery: Reduction and Postmastectomy Reconstruction

Andrea L. Pusic, MD, MHS[a],*, Colleen McCarthy, MD, MSc[a], Stefan J. Cano, PhD[b], Anne F. Klassen, DPhil[c], Carolyn L. Kerrigan, MD[d]

- Study designs used in previous studies
  Case reports and case series
  Cohort studies
  Randomized clinical trials
- Measurement of outcomes
  Traditional outcome measures
  Patient-reported outcome measures
  PROM development and validation

The importance of rigorous measurement
New directions in measurement
- Evaluation of clinical relevancy
  The evidence-based surgery approach
  Efficacy, effectiveness, and efficiency
  Pressures to provide higher levels of evidence
- Acknowledgments
- References

In the current environment of quality surveillance, rapidly evolving surgical techniques, and health care industry restrictions, there is rising pressure on plastic surgeons to provide credible evidence on the effectiveness and efficiency of their surgical practices. This is particularly true for breast reconstruction and reduction surgery. As surgeons, we are increasingly expected to demonstrate the success of our outcomes in a rigorous fashion to health care payers. To satisfy this demand, and to advocate for our patients, we require scientifically rigorous, clinically meaningful data to demonstrate the positive impact of breast surgery on patient quality of life (QOL). The advancement of surgical techniques similarly requires high-level evidence. In the last decade, entirely new breast surgery techniques have evolved. What remains unclear is whether or not these new procedures, some of which carry additional surgical risk and cost, are actually superior from a patient perspective.

Consequently, to support clinical care, research efforts, and advocacy, it is essential that a strong evidence base be established in breast surgery. This article provides an overview of the strengths and weaknesses of different study designs used to address important issues in breast reduction and reconstruction, the appropriateness of different types of outcome measures and measurement tools used to evaluate these outcomes, and the clinical relevancy of establishing a strong evidence base in

---

[a] Memorial Sloan-Kettering Cancer Center, 1275 York Avenue, New York, NY 10021, USA
[b] University College London, Glower Street, London WC1E 6BT, United Kingdom
[c] Department of Pediatrics, McMaster University, Institute of Applied Health Sciences Building, Room 408D, 1400 Main Street West, Hamilton, Ontario L8S 1C7, Canada
[d] Dartmouth-Hitchcock Medical Center, One Medical Center Drive, Lebanon NH 03755, USA
* Corresponding author.
E-mail address: pusica@mskcc.org (A.L. Pusic).

breast surgery. Table 1 includes a glossary of terms that are used in this field and throughout this article.

Study designs used in previous studies

Hierarchies of evidence have been developed to help describe the quality of evidence that may be used to answer clinical research questions [1]. (see the articles in this issue by Sprague, McKay, and Thoma; Haines, McKnight, Duku, Perry, and Thoma; and Thoma, Sprague, Temple, and Archibald). This article considers specific breast surgery study examples and reflects on the limitations and strengths of the study designs used.

Table 1: **Glossary of terms**

Glossary of terms	
Conceptual framework	The expected relationships of items within a domain and of domains within a PRO concept. The validation process confirms the conceptual framework. When used in a clinical trial, the observed relationships among items and domains will again confirm the conceptual framework.
Confounder	An extraneous variable that affects the dependent variables in question but has not been controlled for. The confounding variable can lead to a false conclusion that the dependent variables are in a causal relationship with the independent variable.
Domain	A discrete concept within a multidomain concept. All the items in a single domain contribute to the measurement of the domain concept.
Equipoise	A genuine uncertainty on the part of the expert surgical community about the comparative therapeutic merits of each arm of a clinical trial. (World Medical Association, Declaration of Helsinki. 1964, revised 1996, para. II.3).
Instrument	A means to capture data (eg, questionnaire, diary) plus all the information and documentation that supports its use. Generally, that includes clearly defined methods and instructions for administration or responding, a standard format for data collection, and well-documented methods for scoring, analysis, and interpretation of results.
Item	An individual question, statement, or task that is evaluated by the patient to address a particular concept.
Patient-reported outcome (PRO)	Any report coming directly from patients (ie, study subjects) about a health condition and its treatment.
Patient-reported outcome measures (PROMs)	Questionnaires that quantify health-related quality of life or other significant outcome variables from the patient's perspective.
Psychometric	Psychometrics is the field of study concerned with measurement of differences in traits, such as knowledge, abilities, and personality between individuals and groups of individuals.
Quality of life	A general concept that implies an evaluation of the impact of all aspects of life on general well being.
Questionnaire	A set of questions or items shown to a respondent to get answers for research purposes.
Scale	The system of numbers or verbal anchors by which a value or score is derived. Examples include visual analog scales, Likert scales, and rating scales.
Score	A number derived from a patient's response to items in a questionnaire. A score is computed based on a prespecified, validated scoring algorithm and is subsequently used in statistical analyses of clinical study results. Scores can be computed for individual items, domains, or concepts, or as a summary of items, domains, or concepts.
Validation	The process of assessing a PROMs ability to measure a specific concept or collection of concepts. This ability is described in terms of the instrument's measurement properties that are derived during the validation process. At the conclusion of the process, a set of measurement properties is produced that are specific to the specific population and the specific form and format of the PROM tested.

Adapted from US Department of Health and Human Services. Guidance for industry: patient-reported outcome measures: use in medical product development to support labeling claims: draft guidance. Health Qual Life Outcomes 2006;4:79.; February 2006.

Case reports and case series

While case reports and case series may be considered lower-level evidence [2,3], they have a defined, albeit limited role to play. More specifically, they can be used to generate hypotheses, communicate rare events, and provide descriptive reports, which may be useful when defining or modifying existing surgical techniques. In breast reconstruction, for example, the first case series of deep inferior epigastric perforator (DIEP) flaps [4] provided an important catalyst for other surgeons to begin evaluating this technique [5,6]. While this case series did not provide high-level evidence regarding the efficacy of the procedure, it provided an important springboard for other clinical researchers. It follows that there is no reason to limit innovation or experimentation by restricting the publication or production of case reports; nevertheless, when a new technique is conceived, it should be tested under controlled conditions to generate evidence for its efficacy before being widely disseminated. This methodologic rigor will ultimately serve to limit the possibility that a potentially inferior treatment will replace a superior one simply for reasons of novelty or peer pressure.

Cohort studies

A cohort study "involves identification of two groups (cohorts) of patients, one that receives an exposure of interest, and one that receives a different exposure or no exposure at all. Groups are then followed forward in time to determine outcome" [7,8]. In breast surgery, the "exposure" may be considered the procedure, or aspects thereof. For example, patients having undergone vertical reduction mammoplasty might be separated from those who underwent Weiss pattern reduction, and their outcomes compared at some point after surgery.

In breast surgery, cohort studies play a uniquely important role. In breast reconstruction surgery, many researchers would consider a randomized trial between implant and autologous tissue reconstruction to be unfeasible and perhaps unethical, as it would deny women choice in the method of reconstruction. In this scenario, a well-designed cohort study may be invaluable. Cohort studies also may offer increased generalizability. For example, they may be performed in a manner that effectively mirrors the practice patterns of community plastic surgeons. Because of this, their findings may ultimately be more meaningful to such surgeons and their patients.

The Michigan Breast Reconstruction Outcome Study (MBROS) is an example of a clinically relevant and generalizable, prospective cohort study. This multicenter study evaluated the results of postmastectomy reconstruction from 1994 to 1998. More specifically, a cohort of women who underwent expander-implant breast reconstruction were compared with women who underwent transverse rectus abdominis musculocutaneous (TRAM) flap reconstruction. Patient cohorts who underwent immediate versus delayed reconstruction were similarly compared. Significant procedure type and timing differences were noted across multiple domains, including patient satisfaction, complications, psychosocial function, quality of life, body image, postoperative pain, and physical function [9–13]. The MBROS outcome data have since been used in the creation of a patient decision-making Web site to educate and empower patients considering reconstruction.

In breast reduction surgery, prospective cohort studies have similarly been performed and have provided important data for patient advocacy and negotiations. The Breast Reduction Assessment: Value and Outcomes study was a 9-month, multicenter study, which prospectively examined complications and QOL [14–16]. Using a panel of patient-reported outcome measures (PROMs), the investigators prospectively evaluated a cohort of 179 women undergoing breast reduction surgery. Matched preoperative and postoperative data sets were obtained. In addition, a control cohort was selected which included 88 women with breast hypertrophy and 96 controls. The results of this study demonstrated the ineffectiveness of conservative, nonsurgical measures in treating these patients. Most importantly, the study provided high-level evidence to establish the negative impact of breast hypertrophy, and the benefits of breast reduction surgery, on patients' QOL. Other researchers have subsequently performed a similar prospective evaluation of the QOL following breast reduction surgery. A recent study at McMaster University confirmed the benefits of reduction mammoplasty and the lack of justification for on-going denials of third-party payments, based on patient body mass index [17]. Taken together, such prospective cohort studies with consistent results provide strong evidence upon which patient advocacy efforts may be built.

The main limitation of such cohort studies is the potential for selection bias. Selection bias refers to a systematic difference in characteristics between those who are selected for the intervention group and those who are selected for the comparison group. As an example, patients selected to undergo vertical reduction mammoplasty may have smaller breast volumes than those undergoing Wise-pattern reductions. It is thus essential that breast volume, a potential confounder, be considered when designing such a cohort study. Specifically, patients in the two surgical groups may be matched on the basis of breast volume to minimize selection bias and confounding.

Randomized clinical trials

Randomized controlled trials (RCTs) and systematic reviews of RCTs provide the most rigorous way to determine whether a cause-effect relationship exists between surgical treatment and outcome, and to assess the cost-effectiveness of a procedure. Other study designs, including prospective cohort studies, can detect associations between an intervention and an outcome; however, as described above, they cannot rule out the possibility that the association was caused by a third factor or confounding variable. Instead, by randomly allocating patients to different treatment groups in an RCT, the risk that systematic differences exist between patient groups is minimized [18–20].

In spite of the importance of RCTs, few such studies have been performed among either breast reduction or reconstruction patients. A search of the PubMed database from 1976 to 2007 reveals only 10 RCTs in breast reconstruction [21–30]. Interestingly, the earliest of these was arguably the most significant [30]. In 1982, 64 women were randomized to receive either immediate or delayed breast reconstruction. Using patient-reported outcome measures with known psychometric properties, the investigators reported significantly less psychosocial morbidity among the immediate reconstruction group. Published in the *Lancet* journal, this important study thus established the benefits of immediate reconstruction at a time when delayed reconstruction was the standard of care.

In breast reduction surgery, RCTs have provided insight into a number of important clinical issues. Several studies have, for example, shown that the routine use of drains is of no benefit [31–33]. In the United Kingdom, Iwuagwu and collegues evaluated the effect of breast reduction surgery on multiple patient parameters, including lung function, upper limb nerve conduction, depression, and psychosocial functioning [34–36]. The investigators showed a significant difference in psychosocial functioning between reduction patients and controls. They note that improved lung function correlated with the volume of the reduction. Investigators have also considered the relative merits of vertical breast reductions compared with inferior pedicle or Wise pattern surgery. Cruz-Korchin [31], in a randomized trial of 208 women, found greater patient satisfaction among vertical reduction patients, but a higher rate of revision surgery. This issue of "optimal surgical technique" for breast reduction surgery remains controversial and is currently being studied in an ongoing randomized trial at McMaster University in Ontario, Canada. The study, which will be completed in 2009, will provide further guidance to surgeons as they seek to optimize patient outcomes and satisfaction with the results of reduction mammoplasty (Dr. Achilles Thoma, Personal communication, 2007).

In spite of their very significant strengths, there are a number of reasons why outcome researchers in breast surgery may be hesitant to perform randomized trials (see the article by Thoma, Sprague, Temple, and Archibald in this issue) [37–40]. Specifically, surgeons may feel that it is ethically unsound to enroll patients in a clinical trial when they believe, based on anecdotal or lower level evidence, that one surgical technique is superior to the other. Ethical principles require that there be genuine uncertainty within the expert medical community—not necessarily on the part of an individual investigator—about the preferred treatment. Under such circumstances, it is ethical to offer patients entry in a trial. Such surgical equipoise is abound in breast surgery: Is there a clinically significant difference in donor site morbidity following pedicled TRAM flaps, free TRAM flaps or DIEP flaps? Does the maintenance of breast shape following reduction mammoplasty differ based on the technique performed? Does using AlloDerm in implant-based breast reconstruction improve patient outcomes, and is it cost effective? Do venous couplers minimize the risk of venous thrombosis in microvascular breast reconstruction? The answers to these clinical questions, where genuine uncertainty exists in regards to their answers, can best be answered by RCTs, while meeting the requirements for surgical equipoise.

In some circumstances, an RCT may be ethical but unfeasible because of recruitment difficulties. Indeed, strong patient preferences may also limit recruitment and bias outcomes if not accommodated within the study design. The current controversy regarding DIEP flaps, compared with traditional free and pedicled TRAM flaps, exemplifies this situation. Based on low level or anecdotal evidence, patients and their advocacy groups may perceive that the DIEP flap has an established superiority. In spite of the controversy that exists in the plastic surgery academic literature, patients may thus resist recruitment into a clinical trial in which they would be randomized to either a DIEP flap or traditional TRAM.

Measurement of outcomes

Traditional outcome measures

While an RCT can provide the strongest evidence of the efficacy of an intervention, clinically meaningful, scientifically sound outcome measures are also required if the true impact of the procedure is to be evaluated. Traditional measures of success in breast surgery have focused on complications data, patient photos, and surgeon assessment [41]. While these data remain important, they are no longer sufficient on their own. Research efforts that evaluate outcomes from a surgeon's perspective fail to appreciate that the patient's viewpoint may be substantially different. In breast surgery, it is not uncommon for the surgeon to report an "excellent" result, while the patient remains dissatisfied. Thus, clinical outcomes research in breast surgery must increasingly reflect the importance of issues pertaining to patient satisfaction and quality of life.

Patient-reported outcome measures

In both breast reduction and reconstruction, surgeons endeavor to satisfy their patients with respect to aesthetic results, body image, and QOL. Clinical outcomes research reflects this effort and is increasingly focused on evaluating patient perceptions of outcome.

To appropriately measure the impact of surgically relevant outcomes, well-developed and validated patient questionnaires are needed. Patient questionnaires that are not formally developed or tested (ad hoc questionnaires) may pose reasonable questions, but unless they are psychometrically tested, we cannot be confident about their reliability (ie, ability to produce consistent and reproducible scores) or validity (ie, ability to measure what is intended to be measured).

In the absence of validated instruments specific to breast surgery, many studies use generic instruments. A generic instrument is a broad-based questionnaire, such as the SF-36, that measures health-related QOL in diverse patient populations [42]. While such instruments may be reliable, they may not be sensitive enough to measure changes as a result of surgical intervention or to capture all aspects of outcome specific to breast surgery. The appropriateness of an instrument designed to measure change over time is determined not only by its reliability and validity, but also its responsiveness (ie, sensitivity to change). To evaluate the efficacy of an intervention, such as breast reduction or reconstruction, the instrument must be calibrated to detect a difference after the surgical intervention.

An operative procedure that preserves or improves breast appearance produces changes that can affect multiple spheres of function—or domains—that are related to QOL: not only body image, but also physical, psychologic, and sexual functioning. Instruments that are limited to just one domain, such as aesthetic appearance, may not capture the entirety of the changes that occur after breast surgery. For example, an instrument designed to detect a difference in aesthetic outcome will not be able to measure change in a patient's sense of sexual desirability or femininity. To correctly identify and measure these various dimensions, it is necessary to develop a surgery-specific instrument that considers multiple domains.

A systematic review of breast surgery-specific patient-reported outcome measures identified only seven instruments that had undergone any degree of development and validation in a breast surgery population [43]. Of these seven measures, two were designed for breast reconstruction patients (the MBRS Satisfaction Questionnaire and Body Image Questionnaire) and one for breast reduction patients (the Breast-Related Symptoms Questionnaire or BRSQ) (Table 2). The remaining four addressed the concerns of breast augmentation patients. Upon more rigorous examination, six of the seven measures were not appropriately developed or properly validated, according to the criteria of the Medical Outcomes Trust [48]. Based on this evaluation, their use could not be recommended without reservations [43]. Only the BSRQ, showed evidence of adequate development and validation. Nevertheless, it had significant content limitations. For example, while the BRSQ measured breast reduction symptoms, it failed to address other domains, such as aesthetics and body image.

An additional oncologic breast surgery measure has also recently been published (see Table 2). The Body Image after Breast Cancer Questionnaire (BIBCQ) is a 53-item questionnaire that assesses the long-term impact of breast cancer on body image [47]. There are six domains: vulnerability, body stigma, limitations, body concerns, transparency, and arm concerns. Like the BRSQ, the BIBCQ is a well-developed measure that has undergone appropriate psychometric analysis. However, focusing primarily on body image after mastectomy and lumpectomy, the BIBCQ is weaker when evaluating aesthetic issues after breast reconstruction.

PROM development and validation

To optimally measure QOL in plastic surgery, PROMs should ideally undergo careful and extensive development and psychometric evaluation. Cano and colleagues [49,50] have previously developed PROMs for plastic surgery, based upon current gold standard guidelines in terms of a rigorous, three-stage method for health outcomes instrument development. This approach includes step-by-step procedures for item generation, item reduction, and psychometric evaluation.

Table 2: Patient reported outcome measures developed and validated for use in breast surgery (reduction and reconstruction)

Instrument	Studies describing instrument	What does this scale measure?	Validity	Reliability: 1. Cronbach's α 2. ICC	Responsiveness to change: 1. ES 2. SRM 3. MID
BRSQ	Kerrigan and colleagues, 2001 [14] Kerrigan and colleagues, 2002 [10] Thoma and colleagues, 2005 [44]	Symptoms after breast reduction	Construct validity: statistically significant positive Pearson correlations with SF-36 (Physical) and MBSRQ-AS.	1. Not available 2. 0.87–0.99	1. 3.43 2. 3.28 3. 45.05
MBROS–S	Alderman et al., 2000 [45]	Patient satisfaction after breast reconstruction	Construct validity: Tested using factor analysis models.	1. 0.90 2. Not available	Not available
MBROS–BI	Wilkins et al., 2000 [46]	Patient perceptions of physical appearance after breast reconstruction	Validated in the course of the MBROS study. No formal statistical analysis of validity.	1. 0.89 2. Not available	Not available
BIBCQ	Baxter et al., 2006 [47]	Long-term impact of breast cancer on body image in six domains: vulnerability, body stigma, limitations, body concerns, transparency, and arm concerns	Criterion validity: limited reliability in noncancer control (α = 0.50); 5 of 6 domains nonsignificant in cancer versus control groups. Construct validity: moderate to strong Spearman correlations found between BIBCQ and MBSRQ, IES, RSE, BDI and EORTC QLQ-30	1. 0.77 2. 0.77–0.87	Not available

Abbreviations: BDI, Beck depression index [47]; BIBCQ, Body Image After Breast Cancer Questionnaire [47]; BRSQ, Breast Related Symptoms Questionnaire [10,14,44]; ESI, effect size index (score one day before surgery–score six months after surgery)/standard deviation baseline scores; EORTC QLQ-30, European Organization for Research and Treatment of Cancer – quality of life [47]; ICC, intraclass correlation coefficient; IES, impact of event scale [47]; MBROS–BI, Michigan Breast Reconstruction Outcome Study–body image [46]; MBROS–S, Michigan Breast Reconstruction Outcome Study–satisfaction [45]; MID, minimum important difference; RSE, Rosenberg self-esteem [47]; SRM, standardized response mean (mean change scores/standard deviation of change scores).

As an example of how this process may be performed, the authors of this article recently developed the BREAST-Q, a new PROM that measures satisfaction and QOL among breast reconstruction, breast reduction, and breast augmentation patients. In phase I, the conceptual model and preliminary items were developed from in-depth patient interviews (n = 48) and focus groups, in combination with expert opinion and literature review. In this process, patient input was the predominant component. Pilot testing was also performed to clarify ambiguities in the wording of items, confirm appropriateness, and determine acceptability and completion time. In phase II, extensive multicenter field-testing was performed (n=1992, response rate 70%). Questions are eliminated or revised according to tests of item redundancy, endorsement frequencies, missing data, factor analysis, and tests of scaling assumptions. In this phase, approximately half of the preliminary items were thus eliminated. The remaining items were grouped according to scales, with each scale representing a single aspect of the overall multidimensional conceptual model (examples of scales: satisfaction with breasts, psychosocial well-being, physical well-being, sexuality). In phase III, the BREAST-Q is being administered to large populations of patients to confirm targeting, reliability, convergent and discriminant validity, and responsiveness. It is important to note that this final phase III work may be considered as an on-going process, which may be performed in conjunction with other hypotheses-driven outcomes studies.

The BREAST-Q will provide essential information about the impact and effectiveness of breast surgery from the patients' perspective. With a procedure-specific, modular structure (reconstruction, reduction, and augmentation), it addresses multiple aspects of the patient's experience. Through a meticulous development process, involving both patients and clinicians, content and face validity have been assured. As its content was primarily derived from individual patient interviews, it is conceptually grounded in patient perceptions and highly clinically meaningful. Each BREAST-Q module is designed with pre- and postoperative versions. Compared with other breast-surgery measures previously discussed (see Table 2), the BREAST-Q will thus be uniquely sensitive to surgical change. As such, it will be an important tool to support multicenter research and clinical trials, while also facilitating an evidence-based approach to the management of individual breast surgery patients.

The importance of rigorous measurement

To ideally measure breast surgery outcomes, a PROM must be both clinically meaningful and scientifically sound [51,52]. Scientific soundness refers to the psychometric properties of the measure. Understanding the psychometric properties of a questionnaire is analogous to understanding the calibration and precision of any other measurement device, such as a laboratory scale or temperature gauge. To ensure rigor in measurement, PROMs are thus evaluated and their psychometric properties reported. In the last decade, a series of texts and articles have been published on the subject of methodologic issues regarding PROMs for use in QOL research [53,54], and specifically in relation to plastic surgery [55–57]. At a minimum, measures should be considered with respect to reliability, validity, and responsiveness.

Reliability

Reliability is an important property of a PROM, because it is essential to establish that any changes observed in patient groups are caused by the intervention or disease, and not by problems in the measure. In general, there are two approaches commonly used to evaluate the reliability of rating scales: internal consistency and test-retest reproducibility.

Internal consistency is a function of the number of items and their covariation within a PROM measuring a construct (eg, satisfaction with breast appearance after reconstruction). Cronbach's coefficient alpha [58] is the most commonly used method to estimate internal consistency.

Test-retest reproducibility assesses whether a measure yields the same results on repeated applications when respondents have not changed on the construct being measured [59]. As an example, an investigator might assess a woman's body image 12 months after breast reconstruction surgery. In the absence of any intervention, a repeat assessment at 2 weeks or 1 month later should yield a similar score. The intraclass correlation coefficient (ICC) is the usual statistic computed to estimate test-retest reliability [60].

Validity

Validity is the extent to which an instrument measures what it intends to measure [61–63]. There are two main types of validity that are particularly relevant to instrument development: content validity and construct validity.

Content validity refers to how well a measure covers all the relevant or important issues that pertain to the measure's intended purpose. This is closely related to face validity, which simply indicates whether on not, on the face of it, the measure appears to be assessing the important content grounds. To evaluate content and face validity, qualitative methods are used, as opposed to statistical criteria, using evidence (eg, literature, breast surgeon expert opinion, patient views) obtained during the development of the measure.

Construct validity is evaluated by hypothesizing how a measure should perform and then testing these hypotheses [59]. One of the most common ways to assess this in health measurement is through convergent and discriminant validity. The former offers convergent evidence that the measure is related to other measures (or other variables) of the same construct and the latter provides discriminant evidence that the measure is not related to other distinct constructs [64,65]. Unfortunately, in health measurement it is rare to find a perfect gold standard measure against which to evaluate the validity of a new measure. Furthermore, no single observation can prove the construct validity of a new measure; rather, it is necessary to build up a picture from a broad pattern of relationships of a new measure with other variables [61,63]. Determination of construct validity is thus an ongoing process for both new and well-established measures.

Responsiveness
Responsiveness can be considered as the ability of a measure to detect significant change [60]. In breast reduction and reconstruction surgery, this is particularly critical as plastic surgeons seek to measure the magnitude of the change from the preoperative to postoperative state. Responsiveness is reflected by the magnitude of the standardized change score [66]. There are generally two main approaches to measuring responsiveness: distribution-based approaches, such as the effect size [67] (ie, mean change plus standard deviation), which is interpreted using Cohen's benchmarks for small (less than 0.2), medium (0.5), and large (greater than 0.8) effects [68], and anchor-based approaches, which use an external standard (such as patient judgment about change) and can be interpreted in relation to the minimally important difference (MID) [69,70].

New directions in measurement
Traditionally, PROMs have been developed and evaluated using a measurement theory called classical test theory (CTT) [48,71]. As a means to increase the clinical utility of new questionnaires for individual patients, Rasch measurement [72] and item response theory (IRT) [73] methods are now being increasingly used in PROM development. Fundamentally, these methods differ from CTT, as their focus is the relationship between a person's measurement and their probability of responding to an item, rather than the relationship between a person's measurement and their observed scale total score. This leads to the legitimate summing of items to produce total scores, and in turn the total scores produce interval-level measures from ordinal level rating scale data [74,75]. This improves the accuracy with which investigators can measure clinical change. In addition, these methods provide estimates for patients (and items) that are independent of the sampling distribution of items (and patients). Among other benefits, this allows for accurate estimates suitable for individual person measurement, which can directly inform patient management and treatment. Other advantages include the possibility for item banking, scale equating, computerized scale administration, and methods for handling missing data [76–78]. The BREAST-Q, described above, has been developed using both CTT and IRT methods, and thus offers these important advantages in the measurement of breast surgery outcomes for both clinical and research purposes.

Evaluation of clinical relevancy
The evidence-based surgery approach
The goal of evidence-based surgery is to "integrate individual clinical expertise and the best external evidence" [79]. In breast surgery, this demands the "conscientious, explicit and judicious" use of the best levels of evidence in the care of the individual patient [7,37]. Whatever method of evaluation is deemed appropriate, good study design remains critical to minimizing bias. Lessons learned from RCTs can be applied to other study designs and can help improve the quality of prospective studies and retrospective research. As with RCTs, analyses can adopt inclusion and exclusion criteria, perform sample size calculations before outcome analyses, match participants for prognostic variables, and use statistical modeling to adjust for the effect of confounding.

For plastic surgeons who seek to practice evidence-based breast surgery, a number of guides have been written which provide a checklist approach to study evaluation [80]. Such reviews help clinicians critically examine the evidence and adjust their practices accordingly. In breast reconstruction and reduction surgery, many clinical issues may be resolved by such review. As an example, for a patient undergoing breast reduction, a surgeon may wish to examine the evidence for or against the routine use of drains. For a patient with a Latissimus Dorsi flap reconstruction, the use of quilting sutures at the donor site might be considered. Regarding both of these issues, good quality studies are available and a clinical question can be confidently answered [32,81]. There are, nevertheless, an equal or greater number of other important breast surgery questions that cannot yet be answered from an evidence-based surgery perspective. For these issues, clinically relevant, high-level evidence is still lacking.

Efficacy, effectiveness, and efficiency

Surgical efficacy is a measure of the benefit of a procedure for a given problem under ideal conditions. This is in distinction to effectiveness, which considers the benefit on the intervention under usual or real world conditions. Finally, efficiency refers to the relationship between the success of the intervention and costs [7]. The current controversy surrounding perforator flap versus TRAM flap reconstruction reveals the importance of all three issues. In high volume microsurgical centers, outcomes studies of DIEP flap breast reconstruction have been largely positive [4,6]. This reflects the efficacy of the procedure. What has been less well studied is the outcome of the procedure in low volume centers with more limited microvascular experience. As many women undergo reconstruction in community hospitals, consideration of the effectiveness of the technique is warranted. Finally, given current health care budgetary restriction, cost is a crucial issue. In both the Canadian and American health systems, the efficiency of the DIEP flap relative to the free TRAM has been demonstrated [82,83].

Pressures to provide higher levels of evidence

Breast surgeons need to understand the importance of levels of evidence for a number of reasons. Patient advocacy is one reason. In North America and Europe, it is remains difficult for patients to obtain access to reduction and reconstruction procedures. To advocate for patients, scientifically rigorous data is needed to demonstrate how breast surgery positively impacts on patient QOL. Second, the advancement of surgical techniques requires high-level evidence data. In the last 10 years, entirely new surgical techniques have evolved. What remains unclear is whether or not these new techniques, some of which carry additional surgical risk and cost, are superior to the old techniques from a patient perspective. Third, the Food and Drug Administration and other regulator bodies are demanding scientifically rigorous data on patient outcomes, as typified by the recent struggle to reintroduce silicone breast implants into the United States market. Fourth, attention to pay-for-performance and quality metrics in health care in the United States is increasing. Health care providers are increasingly expected to demonstrate the success of their patient outcomes in a meaningful fashion to health care payers. Ultimately, those providers who can demonstrate better patient outcomes with reliable and valid data may receive higher reimbursements.

As clinical researchers in breast surgery, we can assume an increased leadership role in producing high quality evidence on the efficacy of our surgical interventions. As we move away from the retrospective reporting of cases and nonrandomized studies, toward prospective, randomized trials, the culture of clinical research in breast surgery will be enhanced. As pressure on resources increases, decision makers in health care are increasingly seeking high-quality scientific evidence to support clinical and health policy choices. Ultimately, legislators are looking to develop performance measures based on evidence, rather than on consensus or commonality of practice. Concomitantly, in the spirit of evidence-based surgery, individual clinicians now seek high-level evidence upon which to base decisions for individual patients. We are thus ever more reliant on clinical research to provide high-level evidence to facilitate clinical decision-making, as well as policy negotiations and advocacy.

Acknowledgments

We acknowledge and thank Tomasz R Kosowski for his contribution to this manuscript.

References

[1] Straus S, Haynes B, Glasziou P, et al. Misunderstandings, misperceptions, and mistakes. ACP J Club 2007;146(1):A8–9.
[2] Michel LA. The epistemology of evidence-based medicine. Surg Endosc 2007;21(2):145–51.
[3] Tebbetts JB. Conclusions not supported by data: a recurring story in breast augmentation publications. Plast Reconstr Surg 2006;118(2):563–5 author reply 565–566; [discussion: 566–7].
[4] Allen RJ, Treece P. Deep inferior epigastric perforator flap for breast reconstruction. Ann Plast Surg 1994;32(1):32–8.
[5] Cheveray PM. Breast reconstruction with superficial inferior epigastric artery flaps: a prospective comparison with TRAM and DIEP flaps. Plast Reconstr Surg 2004;114(5):1077–83 [discussion: 1084–5].
[6] Nahabedian MY, Momen B, Galdino G, et al. Breast reconstruction with the free TRAM or DIEP flap: patient selection, choice of flap, and outcome. Plast Reconstr Surg 2002;110(2): 466–75 [discussion: 476–7].
[7] Centre for Evidence-Based Medicine. Glossary of terms in evidence-based medicine. Available at: http://www.cebm.net/?o=1011. Accessed July 31, 2007.
[8] Sutherland SE. Evidence-based dentistry: part IV. Research design and levels of evidence. J Can Dent Assoc 2001;67(7):375–8.

[9] Alderman AK, McMahon L, Wilkins EG. The national utilization of immediate and early delayed breast reconstruction and the effect of sociodemographic factors. Plast Reconstr Surg 2003; 111(2):695–703 [discussion: 704–5].

[10] Kerrigan CL, Collins ED, Kim HM, et al. Reduction mammaplasty: defining medical necessity. Med Decis Making 2002;22(3):208–17.

[11] Sabel MS, Degnim A, Wilkins EG, et al. Mastectomy and concomitant sentinel node biopsy for invasive breast cancer. Am J Surg 2004;187(6): 673–8.

[12] Wilkins EG, Alderman AK. Breast reconstruction practices in North America: current trends and future priorities. Seminars in Plastic Surgery 2004;18:149–55.

[13] Mullan MH, Wilkins EG, Goldfarb S, et al. Prospective analysis of psychosocial outcomes after breast reconstruction: cross-cultural comparisons of one-year postoperative results. J Plast Reconstr Aesthet Surg 2007;60(5):503–8.

[14] Kerrigan CL, Collins ED, Striplin D, et al. The health burden of breast hypertrophy. Plast Reconstr Surg 2001;108(6):1591–9.

[15] Collins ED, Kerrigan CL, Kim M, et al. The effectiveness of surgical and nonsurgical interventions in relieving the symptoms of macromastia. Plast Reconstr Surg 2002;109(5): 1556–66.

[16] Cunningham BL, Gear AJ, Kerrigan CL, et al. Analysis of breast reduction complications derived from the BRAVO study. Plast Reconstr Surg 2005;115(6):1597–604 [erratum in: Plast Reconstr Surg 2005;116(1):361].

[17] Thoma A, Sprague S, Veltri K, et al. A prospective study of patients undergoing breast reduction surgery: health-related quality of life and clinical outcomes. Plast Reconstr Surg 2007;120(1): 13–26.

[18] Abraham NS. Will the dilemma of evidence-based surgery ever be resolved? ANZ J Surg 2006;76(9):855–60.

[19] Brighton B, Bhandari M, Tornetta P 3rd, et al. Hierarchy of evidence: from case reports to randomized controlled trials. Clin Orthop Relat Res 2003;(413):19–24.

[20] Fung EK, Lore JM Jr. Randomized controlled trials for evaluating surgical questions. Arch Otolaryngol Head Neck Surg 2002;128(6): 631–4.

[21] Hall JC, Willsher PC, Hall JL. Randomized clinical trial of single-dose antibiotic prophylaxis for non-reconstructive breast surgery. Br J Surg 2006;93(11):1342–6.

[22] Daltrey I, Thomson H, Hussien M, et al. Randomized clinical trial of the effect of quilting latissimus dorsi flap donor site on seroma formation. Br J Surg 2006;93(7):825–30.

[23] Temple CL, Tse R, Bettger-Hahn M, et al. Sensibility following innervated free TRAM flap for breast reconstruction. Plast Reconstr Surg 2006; 117(7):2119–27 [discussion: 2128–30].

[24] McCarthy CM, Pusic AL, Disa JJ, et al. Unilateral postoperative chest wall radiotherapy in bilateral tissue expander/implant reconstruction patients: a prospective outcomes analysis. Plast Reconstr Surg 2005;116(6):1642–7.

[25] Loewen P, Lamb S, Clugston P. Randomized, double-blind trial of dolasetron versus droperidol for prophylaxis of postoperative nausea and vomiting in patients undergoing TRAM flap breast reconstruction surgery. Ann Plast Surg 2003;51(5):472–7.

[26] Futter CM, Weiler-Mithoff E, Hagen S, et al. Do pre-operative abdominal exercises prevent postoperative donor site complications for women undergoing DIEP flap breast reconstruction? A two-centre, prospective randomised controlled trial. Br J Plast Surg 2003;56(7):674–83.

[27] Moran SL, Nava G, Behnam AB, et al. An outcome analysis comparing the thoracodorsal and internal mammary vessels as recipient sites for microvascular breast reconstruction: a prospective study of 100 patients. Plast Reconstr Surg 2003;111(6):1876–82.

[28] Brandberg Y, Malm M, Blomqvist L. A prospective and randomized study, "SVEA," comparing effects of three methods for delayed breast reconstruction on quality of life, patient-defined problem areas of life, and cosmetic result. Plast Reconstr Surg 2000;105(1):66–74 [discussion: 75–6].

[29] Brandberg Y, Malm M, Rutqvist LE, et al. A prospective randomised study (named SVEA) of three methods of delayed breast reconstruction. Study design, patients' preoperative problems and expectations. Scand J Plast Reconstr Surg Hand Surg 1999;33(2):209–16.

[30] Dean C, Chetty U, Forrest AP. Effects of immediate breast reconstruction on psychosocial morbidity after mastectomy. Lancet 1983;1(8322): 459–62.

[31] Cruz-Korchin N, Korchin L. Vertical versus wise pattern breast reduction: patient satisfaction, revision rates, and complications. Plast Reconstr Surg 2003;112(6):1573–8 [discussion: 1579–81].

[32] Collis N, McGuiness CM, Batchelor AG. Drainage in breast reduction surgery: a prospective randomised intra-patient trail. Br J Plast Surg 2005;58(3):286–9.

[33] Wrye SW, Banducci DR, Mackay D, et al. Routine drainage is not required in reduction mammaplasty. Plast Reconstr Surg 2003;111(1):113–7.

[34] Iwuagwu OC, Platt AJ, Stanley PW, et al. Does reduction mammaplasty improve lung function test in women with macromastia? Results of a randomized controlled trial. Plast Reconstr Surg 2006;118(1):1–6 [discussion: 7].

[35] Iwuagwu OC, Walker LG, Stanley PW, et al. Randomized clinical trial examining psychosocial and quality of life benefits of bilateral breast reduction surgery. Br J Surg 2006;93(3):291–4.

[36] Iwuagwu OC, Bajalan AA, Platt AJ, et al. Effects of reduction mammoplasty on upper-limb nerve

conduction across the thoracic outlet in women with macromastia: a prospective randomized study. Ann Plast Surg 2005;55(5):445–8.
[37] Thoma A. Challenges in creating a good randomized controlled trial in hand surgery. Clin Plast Surg 2005;32(4):563–73, vii.
[38] Young JM, Solomon MJ. Improving the evidence base in surgery: sources of bias in surgical studies. ANZ J Surg 2003;73(7):504–6.
[39] Offer GJ, Perks AG. In search of evidence-based plastic surgery: the problems faced by the specialty. Br J Plast Surg 2000;53(5):427–33.
[40] McLeod RS. Issues in surgical randomized controlled trials. World J Surg 1999;23(12):1210–4.
[41] Lowery JC, Wilkins EG, Kuzon WM, et al. Evaluations of aesthetic results in breast reconstruction: an analysis of reliability. Ann Plast Surg 1996;36(6):85–6.
[42] Ware JE, Gandek B. Overview of the SF-36 Health Survey and the International Quality of Life Assessment (IQOLA) Project. J Clin Epidemiol 1998;51(11):903–12.
[43] Pusic AL, Chen B, Cano S, et al. Measuring quality of life in cosmetic and reconstructive breast surgery: a systematic review of patient-reported outcomes instruments. Plast Reconstr Surg 2007;120(4):823–37.
[44] Thoma A, Sprague S, Veltri K, et al. Methodology and measurement properties of health-related quality of life instruments: a prospective study of patients undergoing breast reduction surgery. Health Qual Life Outcomes 2005;3:44.
[45] Alderman AK, Wilkins EG, Lowery JC, et al. Determinants of patient satisfaction in postmastectomy breast reconstruction. Plast Reconstr Surg 2000;106(4):769–76.
[46] Wilkins EG, Cederna PS, Lowery JC, et al. Prospective analysis of psychosocial outcomes in breast reconstruction: one-year postoperative results from the Michigan Breast Reconstruction Outcome Study. Plast Reconstr Surg 2000;106(5):1014–25 [discussion: 1026–7].
[47] Baxter NN, Goodwin PJ, McLeod RS, et al. Reliability and validity of the body image after breast cancer questionnaire. Breast J 2006;12:221–32.
[48] Scientific Advisory Committee of the Medical Outcomes Trust. Assessing health status and quality-of-life instruments: attributes and review criteria. Qual Life Res 2002;11(3):193–205.
[49] Cano SJ, Browne JP, Lamping DL, et al. The patient outcomes of Surgery-Hand/Arm (POS-Hand/Arm): a new patient-based outcome measure. J Hand Surg [Br] 2004;29(5):477–85.
[50] Cano SJ, Browne JP, Lamping DL, et al. The patient outcomes of surgery—head/neck (POS-Head/Neck): a new patient-based outcome measure. J Plast Reconstr Aesthet Surg 2006;59(1):65–73.
[51] Streiner DL, Norman GR. Health measurement scales: a practical guide to their development and use. 2nd edition. Oxford (UK): Oxford University Press; 1995.
[52] Cronbach L. Validity on parole: how can we go straight? New Directions for Testing and Measurement 1980;5:99–108.
[53] McDowell I, Newell C. Measuring health: a guide to rating scales and questionnaires. New York: Oxford University Press; 1987.
[54] Nunnally JC, Bernstein IH. Psychometric theory. 3rd edition. New York: McGraw-Hill; 1994.
[55] Fitzpatrick R, Jenkinson C, Klassen A, et al. Methods of measuring health-related quality of life and outcome for plastic surgery. Br J Plast Surg 1999;52(4):251–5.
[56] Cano SJ, Browne JP, Lamping DL. Patient-based measures of outcome in plastic surgery: current approaches and future directions. Br J Plast Surg 2004;57(1):1–11.
[57] Cano SJ, Klassen A, Pusic AL. The science behind quality of life measurement: a primer for plastic surgeons. Accepted for publication.
[58] Cronbach LJ. Coefficient alpha and the internal structure of tests. Psychometrika 1951;16: 297–334.
[59] Hays RD, Anderson R, Revicki DA. Psychometric considerations in evaluating health-related quality of life measures. Qual Life Res 1993;2:441–9.
[60] Deyo RA, Diehr P, Patrick DL. Reproducibility and responsiveness of health status measures. Statistics and strategies for evaluation. Control Clin Trials 1991;12(4 Suppl):142S–58S.
[61] Merrick S. Validity of psychological asessment: validation of inferences from persons' responses and performances as scientific inquiry into score meaning. Am Psychologist 1995;50:741.
[62] Kaplan R, Bush J, Berry C. Health status: types of validity and the Index of Well-Being. Health Serv Res 1976;11:478–507.
[63] Anastasi A. Evolving concepts of test validation. Ann Rev Psychol 1986;37:1–15.
[64] Campbell D, Fiske D. Convergent and discriminant validation by the multi trait-multimethod matrix. Psychol Bull 1959;56:81–105.
[65] Campbell D. Recommendations for APA test standards regarding construct, trait, or discriminant validity. Am Psychol 1960;15:546–53.
[66] Guyatt GH. Measuring change over time: assessing the usefulness of evaluative instruments. J Chronic Dis 1987;40:171–8.
[67] Kazis LE, Anderson JJ, Meenan RF. Effect sizes for interpreting changes in health status. Med Care 1989;27:S178–89.
[68] Cohen J. Statistical power for the behavioural sciences. New York: Academic Press; 1977.
[69] Norman GR, Gwadry S, Guyatt GH, et al. Relation of distribution and anchor-based approaches in interpretation of changes in health-related quality of life. Med Care 2001;39(10):1039–47.
[70] Wright B. A history of social science and measurement. Educational Measurement: Issues Pract 1997;16(4):33–45.
[71] Traub R. Classical test theory in historical perspective. Educational Measurement: Issues Pract 1997;16(4):8–14.

[72] Rasch G. Probabilistic models for some intelligence and attainment tests. Chicago: University of Chicago Press; 1960.
[73] Lord FM, Novick MR. Statistical theories of mental test scores. Reading (MA): Addison-Wesley; 1968.
[74] Wright B, Stone M. Best test design: Rasch measurement. Chicago: MESA Press; 1979.
[75] Wright BD, Linacre JM. Observations are always ordinal: measurements however must be interval. Arch Phys Med Rehabil 1989;70(12): 857–60.
[76] Wainer H, Dorans NJ, Flaugher R, et al, editors. Computerized adaptive testing: a primer. Hillsdale (NJ): Lawrence Erlbaum Associates; 1990.
[77] Revicki DA, Cella DF. Health status assessment for the twenty-first century: item response theory, item banking and computer adaptive testing. Qual Life Res 1997;6(6):595–600.
[78] Linacre MJ, et al. Computer-adaptive testing: a methodology whose time has come. In: Chae S, Kang U, Jeon E, editors. Development of computerised middle school achievement tests. Seoul (South Korea): Komesa Press; 2000.
[79] Sackett DL, Rosenberg WM, Gray JA, et al. Evidence based medicine: what it is and what it isn't. BMJ 1996;312(7023):71–2.
[80] Thoma A, Farrokhyar F, Bhandari M, et al. Users' Guide to the Surgical Literature. How to assess a randomized controlled trial in surgery. Can J Surg 2004;47(3):200–8.
[81] Grover K, McManus P. Randomized clinical trial of the effect of quilting latissimus dorsi flap donor site. Br J Surg 2006;93(12):1563; author reply 1563–4.
[82] Kroll SS, Reece GP, Miller MJ, et al. Comparison of cost for DIEP and free TRAM flap breast reconstructions. Plast Reconstr Surg 2001;107(6): 1413–6 [discussion: 1417–8].
[83] Thoma A, Veltri K, Khuthaila D, et al. Comparison of the deep inferior epigastric perforator flap and free transverse rectus abdominis myocutaneous flap in postmastectomy reconstruction: a cost-effectiveness analysis. Plast Reconstr Surg 2004;113(6):1650–61.

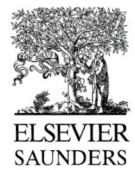

Clinical Research in Head and Neck Reconstruction

Carolyn Levis, MD, MSc, FRCSC[a],*, Stuart Archibald, MD, FRCSC, FACS[b]

- Methodologic challenges in surgical trials
- Study designs
- Cohort studies
- Quality-of-life studies
- Quality-of-life instruments
- Problems and cautions in head and neck surgery quality-of-life studies
- Possible solutions to the head and neck quality of life problems
- References

The National Cancer Institute of Canada reports that malignancies of the head and neck, excluding thyroid, represent 3.5% of new cancers for the year 2007 [1]. Surgery, with or without adjuvant therapy, is frequently used to manage resectable diseases. However, studying the results of surgical treatment is challenging because of the many unique limitations that do not exist to the same degree in other medical fields. There are fundamental differences inherent in the field of surgery that can jeopardize the credibility of surgical research, preventing the work from achieving the highest level of evidence. This may explain the relative paucity of true clinical trials in the surgical literature. Sackett [2] credits Robin McLeod with the most useful report on the management of these challenges for surgical compared with drug trials.

Methodologic challenges in surgical trials

1. **Surgeons learn how to do things better with time.** Given that a learning curve exists for surgical procedures, the number of procedures performed by a surgeon needs to be considered before beginning a randomized controlled trial.
2. **Surgical skills differ among surgeons.** There are implications of differences between surgeons in their expertise in performing different surgeries. It may be that only the best surgeons should be involved in a trial comparing procedures, and they should be allowed to perform the surgery of their choice.
3. **Surgical interventions are difficult to standardize.** Surgeons develop their own modifications and, therefore, all the critical steps of the procedure should be standardized a priori.
4. **Surgeons and patients are not blinded to their surgery.** This is of particular concern when surgeon-measured outcomes, such as complications, or patient-measured outcomes, such as pain, function, or quality of life are used rather than hard outcomes, which can significantly affect the honest reporting of the outcomes.
5. **Patient eligibility may not be determined until after randomization occurs.** The findings at surgery may prohibit a patient from having a procedure (for example, the disease may be too advanced or incorrectly diagnosed).[1]

---

[1] Both 5 and 6 need to be considered when calculating sample size.
[a] Department of Surgery, Division of Plastic and Reconstructive Surgery, St. Joseph's Healthcare, McMaster University, 50 Charlton Avenue East, Room G820, Hamilton, ON L8N 4A6, Canada
[b] Department of Surgery, Division of Otolaryngology–Head and Neck Surgery, St. Joseph's Healthcare, 50 Charlton Avenue East, Room G811, Hamilton, ON L8N 4A6, Canada
* Corresponding author.
E-mail address: levisc@mcmaster.ca (C. Levis).

6. **Time delays between randomization and surgery can affect eligibility.** Unlike drug trials, where patients can be randomized and begin immediately, surgical patients may die from their disease before surgery.[1]
7. **Cointerventions are common in surgical studies.** Nonstandardized perioperative tests, treatments, and consultations that cannot be applied to control patients for reasons of ethics and practicality can affect results.
8. **Recruitment issues can limit surgical trials.** It is usually impossible to limit a new surgery to only patients in a trial (medical trials can allow the use of an otherwise restricted or unreleased drug). Therefore, it may be difficult to recruit enough patients willing to participate in the study. Recruitment issues may be solved with a multicentered surgical trial.

> **Box 1: Levels of evidence—research design rating**
>
> I Evidence from randomized controlled trials
> II-1 Evidence from controlled trials without randomization
> II-2 Evidence from cohort or case-controlled analytic studies, preferably from more than one center or research group
> II-3 Evidence from comparisons between times or places with and without the intervention; dramatic results in uncontrolled experiments could be included here
> III Opinions of respected authorities, based on clinical experience; descriptive studies or reports of expert committees
>
> *Data from* the Canadian Task Force on Preventive Health Care Web site. Available at: www.ctfphc.org

One review of surgical literature listed most reports as case studies or series, and only 7% were randomized, controlled trials, the majority of which compared surgery with a medical therapy [3]. A second review examined the methodology in surgical trials published in 10 prestigious journals over a 6-year period. Several limitations were identified in the 346 articles. Less than 50% of studies reported information about blinding, randomization, and a priori determination of sample size [4].

Despite the shortcomings, it is still imperative to understand the results of surgical treatment to optimize outcomes and provide accurate prognoses. The use of clinical studies in this way is referred to as evidence-based medicine, which assigns the quality of evidence available to assess the risks and benefits of treatments or nontreatment. "Evidence-based medicine is the conscientious, explicit and judicious use of current best evidence in making decisions about the care of individual patients" [5]. Scientific methods of study are used to ensure the best prediction of outcomes of treatment. These methods come in the form of different study designs, which are ranked in a hierarchy of evidence. A commonly used schema in clinical medicine involves five levels based upon the research design, which are ranked according to the degree to which they avoid the various biases (Box 1) (see the article by Sprague, McKay, and Thoma in this issue).

According to most scales, the gold standard of evidence is derived from randomized, double-blind, placebo-controlled trials. High quality studies encompass four discrete principles: (1) well-defined eligibility criteria, minimal missing data; (2) study results should be generalized and applicable to clinical practice; (3) follow-up should be sufficient to permit the outcomes to occur; and (4) statistical power should be adequate to detect differences between a treatment and control [5].

Researchers strive to reach the goal of designing and performing such a trial to test their hypotheses. Despite this evolving concept within medicine as a whole, it has been slow to migrate to modern day surgical practice. A review of the literature on the topic of clinical research in the field of head and neck reconstruction reveals numerous case series and cohort studies, but few clinical trials. These epidemiologic studies report outcomes in terms of function, reconstructive success, incidence of local and regional recurrences, and survival statistics.

An expanding field of research in head and neck surgery and reconstruction is in studying the quality of life in patients diagnosed with cancer and undergoing treatment. These studies focus on the patient's perspective and how they measure success of their treatment, rather than the traditional "hard" endpoints mentioned. Thus, this article reviews study designs, as well as their benefits and limitations, and discusses guidelines that may be considered for future investigation.

Study designs

In simplistic terms, the two main groups of epidemiologic studies are observational and interventions. In both groups, studies can be descriptive or analytic. The main difference is that observation studies identify associations, while analytical studies explore causal relationships. Table 1 depicts the study types that fall within this framework.

True randomized prospective trials (Level I evidence, also termed randomized, controlled trials or RCT) are infrequent in head and neck surgery, and most do not specifically deal with reconstruction. One recent study randomized patients undergoing head and neck cancer resection with free tissue

Table 1: Epidemiologic studies	
Observational (natural experiments)	Intervention (investigator-initiated experiments)
• Descriptive—case reports or series, cross-sectional	• Descriptive—case reports or series
• Analytic—case control or cohort	• Analytic—clinical trial

transfer for reconstruction, to receive low-molecular weight Dextran or aspirin to minimize microvascular thromboses. The treatment did not have an effect on overall flap survival; however, the incidence of systemic complications was significantly related to the method of prophylaxis. The investigators used relative risk to conclude that patients receiving low-molecular-weight Dextran for 120 hours and 48 hours had 7.2 and 3.9 times greater relative risk of developing a systemic complication, respectively, compared with patients receiving aspirin [6].

Other nonreconstruction studies focused their attention on the use of postoperative chemoradiotherapy versus radiotherapy alone for patients with advanced squamous cell carcinoma [7–11]. Four of these studies [7–10] were included in a systematic review, with a meta-analysis to answer the same question regarding combined adjuvant therapy and its ability to improve locoregional control and overall survival, rather than with radiotherapy [12]. If the literature is replete with well-designed and adequately powered RCTs, whose conclusions are corroborative, then the answer is clear regarding the efficacy of the intervention. In cases of disparate results between RCTs (clinical equipoise), or when underpowered from small sample sizes, a meta-analysis is used (see the article by Haines, McKnight, Duku, Perry, and Thoma in this issue).

By pooling the raw data from a group of studies that focus on the same question, more accurate data analysis can be achieved and stronger inferences can be made. The summation of the analysis is typically reported as a standardized measure-of-effect size or a correlation coefficient. Meta-analyses also have limitations. Sources of bias cannot be controlled, and therefore only high quality trials should be included, otherwise a study-level predictor variable must be used to measure the effect of the study quality on the effect size. In addition, only published trials are usually included and therefore, negative effect studies, which are much less likely to appear in the literature, are excluded, which would tend to overestimate the effect size.

This can be overcome by including a calculation that will determine the number of negative studies that would negate the effect. Nevertheless, this type of study can be very useful for a clinical study in surgery, where under powering is a common limitation. Unfortunately, there are no meta-analyses recorded in head and neck reconstructive literature.

Within the field of head and neck surgery, the majority of studies that are largely descriptive in nature are considered "observational." These types of studies identify noncausal associations. There are many case reports and series that describe various characteristics of their population, operative techniques for reconstruction, outcomes and complications, and frequently involve a cohort of patients with cancer of the head and neck with the objective of studying survival and functional outcomes [13,14]. The studies are usually retrospective in nature and typically do not compare different treatments. They also do not address problems that arise from a lack of blinding, randomization, and a priori sample size determination.

It is not the purpose of this article to review all of the studies in head and neck surgery literature, but rather to identify the limitations and challenges that exist by examining certain examples from the literature.

Cohort studies

Numerous series have been published reviewing surgical options and the outcomes of reconstructive procedures for soft tissue and bony defects in the head and neck after ablation. Some series deal with the retrospective, cross-sectional review of certain types of defects and reconstruction [15–19]. For example, Said and colleagues [15] reported on the results of bilobed free osteocutaneous fibula flaps for through-and-through oromandibular defects. The limitations in this study are common to many surgical cohort studies and are reviewed to illustrate the variety of shortcomings. Only 34 subjects were included in the study, which limits the ability to reach statistical significance. It is a reasonable number, however, to identify a trend for some outcomes, such as flap survival. The subjects enrolled were all treated by one surgeon, which has an impact on the generalizability of the study. The results would not be applicable to any other surgeon who is dissimilar to the study surgeon. On a positive note however, when all procedures are performed by one surgeon, certain biases are eliminated that can arise from the differences in the way two or more surgeons perform a procedure. For a prospective study, it would likely be impractical for a single surgeon to enroll enough patients to have adequate power for the study. Therefore, multiple surgeons in several centers should be considered. Moreover, if the surgeon is relatively experienced or works in a tertiary level center, or is subspecialized in the type of surgery being studied, the applicability of the results to a surgeon who has recently entered practice or works in a rural community and is not subspecialized may be very poor. Pooling the results of all surgeons may be misleading, as it fails to identify surgeon-procedure interactions [20]. Many other studies that review defects and the outcomes of reconstruction are plagued by one of the most important challenges in studying head and neck reconstruction: the assessment of the defect. A consistent measure of the defect volume and components is lacking and compromises the ability to compare study subjects.

Another example of a retrospective cohort study in head and neck reconstruction includes an analysis of speech following glossectomy [21]. Forty-one patients from a single center were reviewed 6 months or more after total, subtotal, or partial glossectomy and primary closure, pedicled pectoralis flap major, or free tissue transfer. Adjuvant chemotherapy was used in 10% of patients, while half received radiotherapy either pre- or postoperatively. Despite some strong design techniques in the study, there is concern that there are insufficient numbers in each group to be able to perform any statistical analysis. The investigators employed an analysis of variance to examine the effects of the different variables, and regression analysis was used to further investigate the effects of these factors (use of radiotherapy, extent of resection, method of reconstruction, and presence of lymph note metastasis) on overall speech intelligibility. The results revealed that there was no significant difference in speech scores for patients who had a free flap as reconstruction or primary closure, and patients who were closed with a pectoralis major flap had the poorest speech outcome. The effect of radiation also negatively affected outcome. The method of closure is to some extent dictated by the extent of resection, and in this series the largest defects, leaving the least amount of tongue, were closed with pectoralis major flap, and very small defects were closed primarily. The low numbers in each group hampers the subset analysis. The investigators also considered the effects that time since surgery and timing of radiotherapy would have on speech, but data was not presented in the results. They did however, comment on the tendency for improvement in speech in nonradiated patients between 3 and 12 months postoperatively.

The authors did consider the effect of blinding to some extent, and used nonsurgeons (both naive examiners and speech therapists) to evaluate the speech; however, it was not clearly stated that they were blinded to treatment. One might anticipate that a speech therapist with experience with head and neck cancer patients would be able to determine which patients had more extensive reconstruction, and therefore greater loss of tongue. The assessment of the overall speech intelligibility was measured by three speech therapists, and each scored 10% of the patients a second time 1 week later. This provided inter- and intra-rater reliabilities of 0.95 and 0.97, respectively. Addressing this issue of measurement error is important in a subjective outcome such as speech. As far as the extent of tongue resection, type of reconstruction, and role of radiotherapy, other studies in the literature have addressed speech outcomes in tongue and oral cancer patients speaking other languages with similar results [22–24].

Prospective studies in head and neck surgery are few and most still involve the longitudinal observation of a cohort of patients having had some type of surgery. A recent report was published that prospectively studied swallowing outcome in patients with advanced oral or oropharyngeal cancer, following ablative and free flap reconstructive surgery and adjuvant radiotherapy [25], and confirms results of older studies [26,27]. This study included 80 patients with stage II to IV oral or oropharyngeal squamous cell carcinoma, who underwent composite resection, reconstruction of the defect with free radial forearm flap, and radiotherapy where indicated. Postoperative videofluoroscopic swallowing studies and scintigraphy tests were completed at 6 and 12 months. The swallowing efficiency and the Penetration/Aspiration Scale were analyzed by two experts blinded to the clinical data which, although not stated, presumably means they were unaware of the tumor size, location, history of radiation, and other health conditions. The results indicated that the impairment found at 6 months stabilized to 12 months, and that medical comorbidities, large tumor size, and the involvement of the tongue base and soft palate contributed most to the impairment in swallowing. This article highlights the importance of longitudinal studies in a population where there is great variability in the patients and their disease. Although they do not have the ability to determine causation, repeated measures in the same patient over time excludes the unobserved individual differences between patients.

It is recognized that randomized trials are needed for the evaluation of certain procedures, such as specific cancer surgeries compared with chemo- or radiotherapy protocols. Head and neck surgeons should, however, consider the merits of well-designed, prospective observational studies, with defined outcomes, such as quality of life, as acceptable options [28].

Quality-of-life studies

Surgical treatment always aims to improve the quality of life (QOL) by improving function or form, to reduce troublesome symptoms such as pain, and to improve the overall sense of well-being. Sometimes surgery succeeds in prolonging life by eradicating a disease, but where symptoms dominate the patient's experience, the priority becomes relief of these symptoms where it can be achieved.

Head and neck cancers rank among the most debilitating maladies known, affecting key contributors to a person's sense of well being, such as appearance, speech, and eating; thus, treatment must be directed primarily at improving the patient's function and symptoms, as well as prolonging life. Survival data has shown only a modest incremental improvement over the past 30 years, and major improvements await the development of new treatment approaches. Meanwhile, a significant proportion of patients report that the treatment has been more difficult to endure than the untreated cancer [29,30]. The surgeon's emphasis, therefore, must be on improving the quality of life. Measuring success in this area is difficult, yet all the more imperative to study now that the surgical options for both resections and reconstructions are so numerous.

Procedures are now extensively tailored, in an attempt both to reduce treatment-related morbidity and to maintain oncologic effectiveness. In this, the development of free tissue transfers has afforded much greater scope to change cosmetic and functional outcomes. In light of the observation that one third of the burden of illness is caused by mortality, whereas two-thirds of the burden relates to the quality of life [31], it becomes apparent that head and neck surgeons need to concentrate their efforts on the latter, which matters more to patients who want to return to their preillness level of function, or as close to it as possible. Surgeons now need to become as familiar with the soft data of QOL instruments as they are with the hard end points of survival, local and regional control, tumor response-rates, and laboratory and imaging results, to understand the effectiveness of their treatment.

Quality-of-life instruments

The concept of "health-related quality of life," although intuitive, is nevertheless elusive. What would be "good" quality of life for one person might be "poor" quality for another. Because this cannot be standardized in an absolute sense, the work in this area accepts that the individual patient defines what their own quality of life is from their own perspective. This perspective can be assessed by general or global measures that look at the patient's overall satisfaction with the state of their health and health-related function. Alternatively, it can be measured from the perspective of disease-specific (also known as component) function and the level of patient satisfaction with such function, such as speech or swallowing. Both global definitions and component definitions [32] are relevant in a QOL assessment in head and neck cancer patients. Quality of Life may be defined as "a state of well-being that comprises two components: the ability to perform everyday activities, which reflects physical, psychological, and social well-being; and patient satisfaction with levels of functioning and the control of disease and/or treatment-related symptoms" [33].

Test instruments have been devised and rigorously tested to demonstrate that they meet the criteria of a satisfactory QOL instrument [34], including comprehensibility, reliability, validity, responsiveness, multidimensionality, quantifiability, acceptability, feasibility, and ease of use. Some of these are competing criteria. For instance, an instrument can be designed to be very detailed and sensitive to change, but such a scale may be too lengthy to complete, arduous for sick patients, and may require the assistance of a trained health professional to explain, administer, and score. This will affect its acceptability, particularly if it is to be used repeatedly. Therefore, such a scale may not gain acceptance in clinical practice. This is the case for the Sickness Impact Profile [35].

In many cases, the instruments include general core questions, supplemented by disease or situation-specific modules. Particular attention in the development of these instruments has been paid to the domains studied and the questions within domains, so that the relevant queries are included and unnecessary queries are excluded. This is done so that the tools will have sufficient sensitivity to discriminate between the outcomes, yet avoid obscuring differences in outcomes because of added "noise," which can result from irrelevant queries [36]. QOL tools may be used for their discriminative function (ie, between subject's or group's differences in QOL at a predetermined point in time, as in cross-sectional studies), or for their evaluative function (ie, within subject's or group's differences in QOL over time, as in longitudinal studies) [37]. The most often used instruments in head and neck cancer surgery are listed in Tables 2 and 3. The American Society of Thoracic Surgeons' Web site hosts a quality of life resource

Table 2: General health instruments

Instrument	Scale domains	Citations
American Society of Anaesthesiologists (ASA) score[a]	1–Physical status	[38]
Karnofsky score[b]	1–Health status	[39]
Medical Outcomes Study Short Form 36 (SF-36)	8–Limitations in physical activities, social activities, usual role activities caused by physical health, bodily pain, general mental health, limitation in usual role activities caused by emotional health, vitality, general health perceptions	[40]
Functional Living Index for Cancer (FLIC)	5–Physical well-being and ability, emotional state, sociability, family situation, nausea	[41,42]
Functional Assessment of Cancer Therapy (FACT): General (G)	4–Physical, social and family, emotional, functional well-being	[43]
European Organization for Research and Treatment of Cancer (EORTC) Quality of Life Questionnaire (QLQ) C30	9–Functional scales (physical, role, cognitive, emotional, social), symptom scales (fatigue, pain, nausea, vomiting), global health status, quality-of-life scale, single-item symptom measures	[54]

[a] The ASA score is designed to categorize risk levels for general anesthesia, and involves assessment of co-morbid conditions. Although such conditions impact on overall health status, the score is not directly of QOL. This score may be useful to assess the similarity of the baseline medical condition of pretreatment groups of patients.
[b] The Karnofsky score is a health-worker-derived assessment of a patient's functional performance and is the most widely-used score of this kind. There can be considerable disparity between patient-perceived QOL and Karnofsky performance status scores. For instance, the patient can report a higher QOL than would be measured by the Karnofsky score.

database that lists instruments that have been reported in peer review literature and have published results of reliability and validity (see www.atsqol.org/sections/instruments/index.html).

Typically, a study will use a general measure and a disease-specific measure, sometimes supplementing these with questions around specific function issues. The FACT-G [43] is a self-reported, 28-item general questionnaire, each item scored on a 0 to 4 Likert-type scale. There is an 11-item FACT-H&N [44], similarly scaled and scored. The items are combined, giving six domains of study: physical well being, social and family well being, relationship with physician, emotional well being, functional well being, and head and neck symptoms. The instrument has been used simultaneously on the

Table 3: Disease-specific instruments

Instrument	Scale domains	Citations
Functional Assessment of Cancer Therapy: Head and Neck (FACT-H&N)	6–Physical, social and family, emotional, functional well-being, relationship with doctor, head and neck related symptoms	[44]
Performance Status Scale for Head and Neck (PSS-HN)	3–Normalcy of diet, understandability of speech, eating in public	[45,47]
EORTC Head and Neck (HN)-C35 Module	9–Functional scales (physical, role, cognitive, emotional, social), symptom scales (fatigue, pain, nausea, vomiting), global health status, quality of life scale, single-item symptom measures, specific head and neck specific items	[55]
University of Washington (UW) QOL	3–Physical symptoms, physical functioning, and social function	[48–50]

same patient sample of 151 patients following a variety of treatments for cancers of the larynx (34%), oro- and hypopharynx (35%), and oral cavity (16%) with the PSS-HN, and showed good agreement between them, with each adding to the information provided by the other [45]. The FACT-G and PSS-HN [46] were used in studying the impact of mandibular reconstruction on the QOL in a group of 21 disease-free survivors at 15 months, and showed the QOL and functional results favored mandibular reconstruction over no reconstruction. The PSS-HN [47] was developed to provide a simple yet practical assessment tool, which would measure speech and eating functions, as well as socialization related to those functions. It uses a 5-item subscale for "eating in public" and "understandability of speech" and describes diet according to 10 categories. Each subscale covers the range from normal to maximally impaired. It is administered by health professionals using an unstructured interview, therefore it fits readily into clinic and office visits. It was designed for use with head and neck cancer patients whose disease or treatment affected the oral cavity, pharynx, or larynx, and it has been used widely in QOL studies in head and neck patients.

The University of Washington QOL [48–50] is a self-administered questionnaire designed specifically for head and neck cancer patients to allow standardized QOL comparisons across anatomic subsites and all stages of cancer, and to detect QOL changes over time. It is considered among the easiest questionnaires to administer and covers the domains relevant to head and neck cancer patients, although it is superficial in its direct assessment of mental and emotional issues [51]. It presently consists of 12 categories, with one response required in each from the four or five levels of function described. The 12 categories are: pain, disfigurement, activity, recreation and entertainment, chewing, swallowing, speech, shoulder disability, taste, saliva, mood, and anxiety. Although it lacks a general or core version, there are three additional items, which yield a global score. The instrument has been shown to be highly reliable and valid, with excellent responsiveness to change and excellent acceptance by patients. It tends to be widely used in surgical settings. A recent example of its use was to evaluate 130 oral cancer surgical patients who completed the questionnaire before treatment, then at 6 and 12 months after treatment [52]. The instrument was supplemented with an 11-point clinical examination [53]. The results revealed that the main predictors of cumulative UW-QOL scores were tumor size, clinical functional score, and type of operation, with a fall from preoperative levels of function at 6 months, and a slight improvement by 12 months. Oral function was shown to be a major contributor to QOL in this study.

The European Organization for Research and Treatment of Cancer (EORTC) Quality of Life Questionnaire [54] has also received wide acceptance in both radiation therapy and surgical trials. It is an elaborate instrument, which takes longer to complete than the UW QOL. The instrument is a self-administered questionnaire consisting of a core of thirty questions (C30) evaluating six domains: physical function, role function (work and leisure activities), social function, emotional function, cognitive function, and general health-related QOL, using multi-item scales scored 1 to 100 each, with good function receiving high scores, three multi-item symptom scales (pain, fatigue, and emesis), and six single items (pain, dyspnea, appetite, sleep disorders, diarrhea, constipation, and economic sequelae). The symptom and single items are scored such that good outcomes receive low scores. The head and neck module (HN-35) [55] evaluates symptoms and sequelae of treatment in 35 items, using six multi-item scales covering pain in the head and neck, swallowing, nutrition, speech, social function, and body image, plus seven single items—coughing, feeling ill, use of nutritional supplements, use of pain killers, use of feeding tubes, weight loss, and weight gain—with good outcomes receiving low scores. This instrument explores functional, mental, and emotional issues in depth.

A recent example of how to use QOL instruments successfully is the study by Schliephake and Jamil [56] that evaluated 107 oral cancer surgical patients for the impact of soft tissue reconstruction on function and quality of life. The EORTC QLQ C30 and EORTC HN-C35 were used before treatment and at 3, 6, and 12 months. The extent of the ablative defects and the type of free flap reconstruction affected the QOL scores with the usual decline seen after treatment to 6 months, but a subsequent increase up to 12 months, at which time the radial forearm free flap reconstructed patients had achieved higher QOL scores than they had at baseline. The EORTC H&N is possibly the most robust tool to detect minor changes in speech and swallowing [57]. The power of this scale is corroborated by a recent but as yet, unpublished study that analyzes the reliability, validity, and responsiveness to change in 12 quality of life instruments for head and neck cancer patients (Ayeni, Sollazo, Thoma, et al, unpublished data, 2007).

Any of the above instruments will be helpful in assessing either function or QOL or both. Which instrument to select depends on the question one wishes to answer. More detail of specific functions may be obtained by using supplemental questionnaires [52,58].

Problems and cautions in head and neck surgery quality-of-life studies

Progress in QOL studies in head and neck cancer surgery are hampered by a number of potential problems. The significance of this depends on the question that the study hopes to answer. For instance, for some questions, only a few patients might be required. The following is a list of limitations in head and neck surgery studies:

1. Lack of a uniformly accepted score or system, which would describe the extent of the anatomical defect and physiologic disruption resulting from the various resections. Without such a standardized system, it is impossible to compare the outcomes of various approaches in reconstruction. This may be, perhaps, the most significant limitation.
2. Few patients are available because:
   a. Few patients have cancer of the same head and neck subsite
   b. Only some of these patients have surgery
   c. Reconstruction is not indicated for all surgical patients
   d. Reconstructions of the same type and extent are not common as the permutations of extent of resection and reconstruction are very numerous
   e. Surgeons may refuse to let their patients enter studies
   f. Patients may not consent to participate or may withdraw from a study
   g. Recurrent disease or the development of a new primary cancer, may confound QOL and survival
3. Insufficient sensitivity of the QOL instruments to detect the incremental improvements, which result from innovations in reconstructive surgery in cross-sectional studies, and to detect improvement or deterioration in longitudinal studies [59]
4. Large number of patients may be required to demonstrate significant differences in outcomes [3,58–60]
5. Collecting QOL data places demands on time and scarce resources; this should not be underestimated [59]
6. QOL in disease-free patients typically declines for 3 to 6 months following treatment, then gradually improves for up to 12 months [56]; therefore, patients need to be assessed at similar points after treatment in cross-sectional studies
7. The QOL data tends to be collected in the best-adapting surviving patients, whereas the patients with the lowest QOL are reluctant or too ill to complete questionnaires. This biases the QOL results so that they appear better than they are across all treated patients [61].

Possible solutions to the head and neck quality of life problems

1. Multicenter studies may help overcome the few patients available in any one center. This will be expensive, as it requires an infrastructure to be developed for any trial. Once the pattern is established, subsequent studies should be easier. Another alternative is to provide the raw demographic and staging data, as well as QOL domain scores, in case series publications, so that meta-analysis can eventually be performed.
2. Trials should be designed with QOL outcomes as the primary measure. The other data, such as flap survival, disease-free survival, local and regional control, development of new primary cancers, and disease-specific survival will be collected as well.
3. The development of an accepted system for describing the anatomic and physiologic deficits of resections is very important. Whereas from the oncologic point of view, the site and description of the size of the primary (T-stage, thickness, etc.) may suffice when studying the oncologically relevant outcomes of local and regional recurrence, this is insufficient when attempting to study functional outcomes including QOL.
4. Tracking the patient-derived information on questions around the function of interest, rather than the pooled score for an entire domain, may allow detection of subtle changes in the outcome of interest in a longitudinal study to evaluate a particular innovation in reconstruction. Alternatively, supplemental queries concerning a specific function postoperatively may need to be added to the head and neck disease-specific instrument used, realizing that such additional queries have not been shown to be valid or reliable.

It may still be necessary to develop additional general and disease-specific instruments to assess outcomes in head and neck surgery and reconstruction; however, at this time this cannot be determined. In existing studies, useful systems for measuring the defect sizes are not reported. With the development of a system, which will allow defects to be measured, the results of using the existing scales would become meaningful. Until then, variations in head and neck defects can obscure the changes or differences that are measured by the existing QOL instruments.

Reconstructive head and neck surgery is not unlike other surgical fields in its paucity of clinical research. True randomized and prospective trials are rarely an option for research because of the many challenges and limitations, which have been addressed in this article. The types of studies that make up the head and neck reconstructive literature have been reviewed, as well as the evolution toward the use quality-of-life scales, which measure the patient's satisfaction with their health state and function. Although difficulties exist in the design and execution of surgical studies, head and neck surgeons are encouraged to continue the pursuit of measuring the results of their care.

References

[1] Canadian Cancer Statistics 2007. Toronto: Canadian Cancer Society/National Cancer Institute of Canada; 2007.
[2] Sackett DL. The principles behind the tactics of performing therapeutic trials. In: Haynes RB, Sackett DL, Guyatt GH, et al, editors. Clinical epidemiology: how to do clinical practice research. Philadelphia: Lippincott Williams & Wilkins; 2006. p. 173–243.
[3] Horton R. Surgical research or comic opera: questions but few answers. Lancet 1996;347: 984–5.
[4] Hall JC, Mills R, Nguyen H, et al. Methodologic standards in surgical trials. Surgery 1996;119: 466–72.
[5] Sackett DL, Rosenberg WM, Gray JA, et al. Evidence based medicine: what it is and what it isn't. BMJ 1996;312(7023):71–2.
[6] Disa JJ, Polvora VP, Pusic AL, et al. Dextran-related complications in head and neck microsurgery: do the benefits outweigh the risks? A prospective randomized analysis. Plast Reconstr Surg 2003;112:1534–9.
[7] Bernier J, Domenge C, Ozsahin M, et al. Postoperative irradiation with or without concomitant chemotherapy for locally advance head and neck cancer. N Engl J Med 2004;350:1945–52.
[8] Cooper JS, Pajak TF, Forastiere AA, et al. Postoperative concurrent radiotherapy and chemotherapy for high-risk squamous-cell carcinoma of the head and neck. N Engl J Med 2004;350:1937–44.
[9] Bachaud JM, Cohen-Jonathan E, Alzieu D, et al. Combined postoperative radiotherapy and weekly cisplatin infusion for locally advanced head and neck carcinoma: final report of a randomized trial. Int J Radiat Oncol Biol Phys 1996;36:999–1004.
[10] Smid L, Budihna M, Zakotnik B, et al. Postoperative concomitant irradiation and chemotherapy with mitomycin C and bleomycin for advanced head-and-neck carcinoma. Int J Radiat Oncol Biol Phys 2003;56:1055–62.
[11] Zakotnik B, Budihna M, Smid L, et al. Patterns of failure in patients with locally advanced head and neck cancer treated postoperatively with irradiation or concomitant irradiation with Mitomycin C and Bleomycin. Int J Radiat Oncol Biol Phys 2007;67:685–90.
[12] Winquist E, Oliver T, Gilbert R. Postoperative chemoradiotherapy for advanced squamous cell carcinoma of the head and neck: a systematic review with meta-analysis. Head Neck 2007;9: 38–46.
[13] Rieger JM, Zalmanowitz JG, Li SY, et al. Functional outcomes after surgical reconstruction of the base of tongue using the radial forearm free flap in patients with oropharyngeal carcinoma. Head Neck 2007;29(11):1024–32.
[14] Malone JP, Stephens JA, Grecula JC, et al. Disease control, survival and functional outcome after multimodal treatment for advanced-stage tongue base cancer. Head Neck 2004;26:561–72.
[15] Said M, Heffelfinger R, Sercarz JA. Bilobed fibula flap for reconstruction of through-and-through oromandibular defects. Head Neck 2007;29:829–34.
[16] Deleyiannis FW, Lee E, Gastman B, et al. Prognosis as a determinant of free flap utilization for reconstruction of the lateral mandibular defect. Head Neck 2006;28:1061–8.
[17] Murray DJ, Gilbert RW, Vesely MJ, et al. Functional outcomes and donor site morbidity following circumferential pharyngoesophageal reconstruction using an anterolateral thigh flap and salivary bypass tube. Head Neck 2007;29: 147–54.
[18] Kim Y, Smith J, Sercarz J, et al. Fixation of mandibular osteotomies: comparison of locking and nonlocking hardware. Head Neck 2007;29: 453–7.
[19] Smith RB, Henstrom DK, Karnell LH, et al. Scapula osteocutaneous free flap reconstruction of the head and neck: impact of flap choice on surgical and medical complications. Head Neck 2007;29:446–52.
[20] Reeves B. Health-technology assessment in surgery. Lancet 1999;353(Suppl 1):3–5.
[21] Wong RK, Poon ES, Woo CY, et al. Speech outcomes in Cantonese patients after glossectomy. Head Neck 2007;29:758–64.
[22] Furia CL, Kowalski LP, Latorre MR, et al. Speech intelligibility after glossectomy and speech rehabilitation. Arch Otolaryngol Head Neck Surg 2001;127:877–83.
[23] Shpitzer T, Gur E, Feinmesser R, et al. Transoral reconstruction of the mobile tongue, using radial forearm free flap. Microsurgery 2003;23:18–20.
[24] Haughey BH, Taylor SM, Fuller D. Fasciocutaneous flap reconstruction of the tongue and floor of month. Otolaryngol Head Neck Surg 2002; 128:1388–95.
[25] Borggreven PA, Verdonck-de Leeuw I, Rinkel RN, et al. Swallowing after major surgery of the oral

cavity or oropharynx: a prospective and longitudinal assessment of patients treated by microvaxcular soft tissue reconstruction. Head Neck 2007;29:638–47.
[26] Skoner JM, Andersen PE, Cohen JI, et al. Swallowing function and tracheotomy dependence after combined-modality treatment including free tissue transfer for advanced-stage oropharyngeal cancer. Laryngoscope 2003;113:1294–8.
[27] Su WF, Hsia YJ, Chang YC, et al. Functional comparison after reconstruction with a radial forearm free flap or a pectoralis major flap for cancer of the tongue. Otolaryngol Head Neck Surg 2003;128:412–8.
[28] Meakins JL. Innovation in surgery. Am J Surg 2002;183:399–405.
[29] Burns L, Chase D, Goodwin WJ. Treatment of patients with stage IV cancer: do the ends justify the means? Otolaryngol Head Neck Surg 1987; 97:8–14.
[30] Gamba A, Romano M, Grosso IM, et al. Psychosocial adjustment of patients surgically treated for head and neck cancer. Head Neck 1992;14: 218–23.
[31] Murray D, Lopez A. The global burden of disease: a comprehensive assessment of mortality and disability from diseases, injuries, and risk factors in 1990 and projected to 2020. Boston: World Health Organization, Harvard School of Public Health; 1996.
[32] Fitzpatrick R, Davey C, Buxton MJ, et al. Evaluating patient-based outcome measures for use in clinical trials. Health Technol Assess 1998;2: i–iv, 1–74.
[33] Gotay CC, Moore TD. Assessing quality of life in head and neck cancer. Qual Life Res 1992;1:5–7.
[34] Osoba D. Guidelines for measuring health-related quality of life in clinical trials. In: Hays RD, Fayers PM, Staquet MJ, editors. Quality of life assessment in clinical trials. Oxford (UK): Oxford University Press; 1998. p. 19–35.
[35] Pollard WE, Bobbitt RA, Bergner M, et al. The sickness impact profile: reliability of a health status measure. Med Care 1976;14:146–55.
[36] Karnell LH, Funk GF, Hoffman HT. Assessing head neck cancer patient outcome domains. Head Neck 2000;22:6–11.
[37] Sackett DL, Guyatt GH, et al. Generating outcome measurements, especially for quality of life. In: Haynes RB, Sackett DL, Guyatt GH, editors. Clinical epidemiology: how to do clinical practice research. Philadelphia: Lippincott Williams & Wilkins; 2006. p. 388–412.
[38] ASA Physical Status Classification. In: American Society of Anesthesiologists: handbook for delegates. 1974; 416–32.
[39] Karnofsky DA, Abelmann WH, Craver LF, et al. The use of nitrogen mustards in the palliative treatment of carcinoma. Cancer 1978;1: 634–56.
[40] Ware JE, Sherbourne CD. The MOS 36-item short-form health survey (SF36):I: conceptual framework and item selection. Med Care 1992; 30:473–83.
[41] Schipper H, Clinch J, McMurray A, et al. Measuring the quality of life of cancer patients: the functional living index—cancer: development and validation. J Clin Oncol 1984;2(5):472–83.
[42] Schipper H, Levitt M. Measuring quality of life: risks and benefits. Cancer Treat Rep 1985;69: 1115–23.
[43] Cella DF, Tulsky DS, Gray G, et al. The functional assessment of cancer therapy scale: development and validation of the general measure. J Clin Oncol 1993;11:570–9.
[44] D'Antonio LL, Zimmerman GJ, Cella DF, et al. Quality of life and functional status measures in patients with head and neck cancer. Arch Otolaryngol Head Neck Surg 1996;122:482–7.
[45] List MA, D'Antonio LL, Cella DF, et al. The performance status scale for head and neck cancer patients and the functional assessment of cancer therapy—head and neck scale. Cancer 1996;77: 2294–301.
[46] Wilson KM, Rizk N, Armstrong SL. Effects of hemimandibulectomy on quality of life. Laryngoscope 1998;108:1574–7.
[47] List MA, Ritter-Sterr C, Lansky SB. A performance status scale for head and neck patients. Cancer 1990;66:564–9.
[48] Hassan SJ, Weymuller EA. Assessment of quality of life in head and neck cancer patients. Head Neck 1993;15:485–96.
[49] Weymuller EA, Alsarraf R, Yueh B, et al. Analysis of the performance characteristics of the University of Washington quality of life instrument and its modification (UW-QOL-R). Arch Otolaryngol Head Neck Surg 2001;127:489–93.
[50] Weymuller EA, Yueh B, Deleyiannis FW, et al. Quality of life in head and neck cancer. Laryngoscope 2000;110:4–7.
[51] Rogers SN, Lowe K, Brown JS, et al. A comparison between the University of Washington Head and Neck Disease-Specific Measure and the Medical Short Form 36, EORTC QOQ-C33 and EORTC Head and Neck 35. Oral Oncol 1998;34:361–72.
[52] Rogers SN, Lowe D, Fisher SE, et al. Health-related quality of life and clinical function after primary surgery for oral cancer. Br J Oral Maxillofac Surg 2002;40:11–8.
[53] Rogers SN, Lowe D, Patel M, et al. Clinical function after primary surgery for oral and oropharyngeal cancer: an 11-item examination. Br J Oral Maxillofac Surg 2002;40:1–10.
[54] Aaronson NK, Ahmedzai S, Bergman B, et al. The European Organization for Research and Treatment of Cancer QLQ-C30: a quality-of-life instrument for use in international clinical trials in oncology. J Natl Cancer Inst 1993;85:365–76.
[55] Bjordal K, Hammerlid E, Ahlner-Elmqvist M, et al. Quality of life in head and neck cancer patients: validation of the European Organization for Research and Treatment of Cancer Quality

of Life Questionnaire (QLQ)—H&N35. J Clin Oncol 1999;17:1008–101.

[56] Schliephake H, Jamil MU. Impact of intraoral soft-tissue reconstruction on the development of quality of life after ablative surgery in patients with oral cancer. Plast Reconstr Surg 2002;109: 421–30.

[57] Julious SA, Campbell MJ, Walker SJ, et al. Sample sizes for cancer trials where health related quality of life is the primary outcome. Br J Cancer 2000;83:959–63.

[58] Duncan GG, Epstein JB, Dongsheng T. Quality of life, mucositis, and xerostomia from radiotherapy for head and neck cancers: a report from the NCIC CTG HN2 randomized trial of an antimicrobial lozenge to prevent mucositis. Head Neck 2005;27:421–8.

[59] Weymuller EA, Yueh B, Deleyiannis WB, et al. Quality of life in patients with head and neck cancer. Arch Otolaryngol Head Neck Surg 2000;126:329–36.

[60] Deleyiannis FW, Weymuller EA, Coltrera MD. Quality of life of disease-free survivors of advanced (stage III or IV) oropharyngeal cancer. Head Neck 1997;19:466–73.

[61] Gal TJ, Futran ND. Outcomes research in head and neck reconstruction. Facial Plast Surg 2002; 18:113–7.

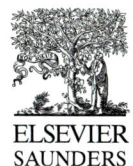

Measuring Outcomes in Hand Surgery

Amy K. Alderman, MD, MPH*, Kevin C. Chung, MD, MS

- National trends surgical care
- Surgical complications
- Objective measures of hand function
- Patient-reported measures of hand function
- Economic burden
- External funding for outcomes research in hand surgery
- The future of outcomes research in hand surgery
- References

In our consumer-driven medical environment, both payers and patients are demanding reliable data that can inform medical decisions and lead to cost-effective medical practices. Anecdotal experience is no longer an acceptable platform for making medical decisions. Patients want more information about surgical outcomes, including information not just about functional recovery. They want to know how satisfied they will be with the delivery of their care, with their psychological and social well-being, and, even in hand surgery, with their aesthetic appearance [1,2]. Outcomes research provides patients with this information by studying the end results of medical practices and interventions that directly affect both the patient and the global health care environment. These end results include a wide range of measurable effects that people experience, such as quality of life (including the ability to function and psychosocial well-being), satisfaction with care, mortality, and economic burden [3,4]. In addition, payers want value. They are demanding cost-effective medical practices based on evidence-based medicine. As a result, outcomes research is providing "report cards" that patients and payers are using to assess the quality of different health plans and providers [3].

The outcomes movement gained strength in the 1980s when John Wennberg and the Dartmouth Atlas of Healthcare discovered the association between geography and health care utilization [5–7]. The rates of common medical procedures, such as hip replacements [8] and hysterectomies [9], varied dramatically by geography despite similar rates of disease. Surprisingly, little data existed to support the health impact of many of these procedures. This revelation inspired researchers to develop tools that can inform patients and providers of the risks and benefits of different health care interventions. It also moved the federal government to develop the Agency for Healthcare Research and Quality, whose mission is to examine how people get access to health care, how much care costs, and what happens to patients as a result of this care. The agency's primary goals are to promote the delivery of high quality medical care, reduce medical errors, and improve patient safety [10].

Section of Plastic and Reconstructive Surgery, Department of Surgery, University of Michigan, The University of Michigan Medical Center, 2130 Taubman Center, 1500 E. Medical Center Drive, Ann Arbor, MI 48109-0340, USA
* Corresponding author.
E-mail address: aalder@umich.edu (A.K. Alderman).

Endpoint measures in outcomes research and the instruments used to evaluate these endpoints are often disease or region specific. Investigators are challenged to use appropriate techniques to measure common endpoints, such as health-related quality of life (HRQL), economic burden, and patient satisfaction, in a reliable and valid manner across multiple health conditions [4]. Ultimately, by linking the care patients receive with their health outcomes, we can better monitor the quality of care for patients. Hand surgery has many different measurable outcomes that can be used to monitor the quality of surgical practice, inform practice guidelines, and aid in the appropriate allocation of health care resources. This article describes examples of research tools available to study surgical outcomes of diseases of the hand and upper extremity.

National trends surgical care

Researchers can monitor quality indicators and identify areas of overuse, underuse, or misuse by studying epidemiological trends in health care delivery. For example, Wennberg [5,6] used the Medicare database to extensively study geographical variations in the use of common surgical procedures. Some areas of the country were identified as having higher than expected rates of common surgical procedures, giving those region a so-called "surgical signature." These unwanted variations in the use of common surgical procedures lead to higher health care costs without improvements in health care quality. Shared medical decision-making and outcomes research have been proposed as promising strategies to reduce regional variations in surgical care [5].

The use of large administrative databases to study epidemiological trends in hand surgery is challenging. The data easiest to abstract are those for mortality. However, such data are not relevant to most diseases of the hand and upper extremity. Even so, national databases can be used to assess regional trends in the surgical care of hand patients. These analyses can assist with the generation of hypotheses that can be further explored at the patient or health system level. For example, the Surveillance and End Results (SEER) database, which is sponsored by the National Cancer Institute, collects medical and surgical data on a national sample of cancer patients. This database can be used to evaluate sociodemographic trends in care [11–13]. For example, in the upper-extremity sarcoma population, significant variations according to patient race were observed in the use of adjuvant radiotherapy. Another national database is the Healthcare Cost and Utilization Project (HCUP), which is sponsored by the Agency for Healthcare Research and Quality. HCUP is an administrative database that collects claims data from multiple payers and has been used to evaluate epidemiological trends in finger replantation [14] and rheumatoid arthritis hand procedures [15]. For rheumatoid arthritis hand surgery, significant variations in surgical care were observed by patient gender and geographical location. The source of these variations were then further explored at patient and physician level through national surveys [2,16,17].

Currently available national databases (Table 1) include SEER for cancer care, the National Surgical Quality Improvement Program sponsored by the American College of Surgeons for general surgical care [18], and HCUP. HCUP includes the Nationwide Inpatient Sample, the State Inpatient Database, the State Ambulatory Surgery Database, the Kids' Inpatient Database, and the State Emergency Department Databases [19]. Medicare has three databases: Medicare Provider Analysis and Review File (inpatient claims), Hospital Outpatient Standard Analytic File (outpatient facility services) and the Physician/Supplier File (physician and other medical services) [20]. The Medicare databases are limited to patients aged 65 years and older. In summary, large database analyses provide a "10,000-feet" view of the health care system and can guide researchers to potential areas of concern that can be investigated more closely at the patient or health system level.

Surgical complications

Surgical complications must be assessed using disease-specific instruments that are measured at the clinically appropriate time interval. Chronic conditions, such as rheumatoid arthritis, may require much longer follow-up assessments [21] compared to those required for traumatic injuries, which tend to be more acute [2]. Surgical complications in hand surgery have historically been evaluated from a single-surgeon retrospective viewpoint [22]. Although this method is cost-effective, the data have limited generalizability to other practice settings. Furthermore, the retrospective study design is subject to biases. Unmeasured factors and reporting bias may influence the study's outcomes. A prospective, randomized controlled clinical trial (RCT) is the benchmark for evaluating surgical outcomes, such as complications and objective measures of physical function. When used in a multicenter design, these studies can provide the most unbiased data for representing surgical outcomes across a variety of practice settings [23]. However, the high costs associated with RCTs often limit their use in hand surgery, resulting in small samples and, subsequently, studies that are underpowered. Regardless of how well a study is designed, an underpowered study will decrease the study's statistical power to find significant differences in treatment outcomes [24,25]. (See the article by Thoma, Sprague, Temple, and Archibald in this issue.)

Meta-analysis is an alternative tool that can be used to address power limitations from studies with small samples. A meta-analysis statistically combines the results from multiple studies that have similar hypotheses [26]. However, the meta-analysis does more than just combine the effect sizes from a set of studies. The analysis can test the null hypothesis and show if more variation is present than what would be expected from sampling different research participants [26,27]. The quality of the meta-analysis is entirely dependent on the quality of the data analyzed. Traditionally, only level one or level two data from RCTs (and occasionally prospective cohort trials) are analyzed in the meta-analysis. This is because the meta-analysis cannot control for potential sources of bias. A good meta-analysis of poorly designed studies will result in a flawed statistical analysis [26]. A systematic review is a summary and appraisal of high-quality health care literature [28–31]. In hand surgery, this approach has been used to assess metacarpophalangeal joint implants in the rheumatoid arthritis population [28], digital sympathectomy for the treatment of chronic digital ischemia [30], the effectiveness of endoscopic versus open carpal tunnel release [32], and the surgical treatment of osteoarthritis of the thumb carpometacarpal joint [33]. The Cochrane Collaboration is the best known source of published systematic reviews of randomized trials [34]. (See the article by Haines, McKnight, Duku, Perry, and Thoma in this issue.)

Objective measures of hand function

Objective measures of hand function provide precise, quantifiable outcomes data. These are by far the most commonly reported outcome measures in hand surgery. These objective measures include measurements for impairment of movement, power, and sensibility [35–38]. So that data are reliable and valid, objective measurement must be performed with calibrated instruments under strict protocols [39]. By using universally available instruments for measurement, researchers can compare functional outcomes among different surgical techniques. For example, the functional outcomes of carpal tunnel surgery have been extensively evaluated by open versus endoscopic surgical technique [32,40,41].

Patient-reported measures of hand function

With the variety of surgical techniques available in hand surgery, choosing the "right" operation can by a daunting task, even for experienced surgeons and highly educated patients. Patient-reported outcome measures can provide patients and physicians with reliable information to assist in this decision-making process. In particular, patient satisfaction and HRQL data offer patients a means of evaluating and comparing options based on the perspectives of previous patients. By comparison, traditional tools, such as a hand radiograph, give little or no insight as to what the patient is experiencing. Patient satisfaction and HRQL data could be useful for a patient thinking about undergoing a new surgical procedure that may provide an additional 10° of finger flexion. The patient may decide that this additional 10° of flexion is not worth the perioperative pain and longer occupational therapy requirements associated with the new procedure. In other words, the patient may conclude that the surgery would result in poorer, not better, quality of life.

Patient-reported measures of health outcomes are gaining recognition in both the local and national health policy arenas. The National Institutes of Health (NIH) in 2004 formed the Patient-Reported Outcomes Measurement Information System, which is aimed at establishing accurate and efficient measurement of patient-reported symptoms and other health outcomes [42]. This NIH initiative, managed by the National Institute of Arthritis and Musculoskeletal and Skin Diseases, is developing measures of patient-reported symptoms, such as pain and other aspects of HRQL, across a wide variety of chronic diseases and conditions [43]. The traditional components of HRQL include three main dimensions of health—physical, mental, and social well-being [36]. The elements of patient satisfaction research include two measurable components: (1) patient satisfaction with the decision-making process for surgery and (2) patient satisfaction with the surgical outcome. Patients can appraise differently their satisfaction with the treatment outcome and the process by which they arrived at a treatment approach.

The shift in emphasis from objective measures to patient-reported measures has led to a surge in questionnaire development. The approach to developing questionnaires for measuring HRQL and patient satisfaction is the basis of social survey research and requires several stages, such as item generation, item reduction, pretesting, field management, and attribute testing [36,44,45].

Instrument development often begins with qualitative research, such as focus groups or qualitative interviews, that informs the conceptual model and construct domains. Focus groups involve interviews with multiple people at once about their attitudes towards the research topic. Questions are structured to facilitate conversation among the participants

Table 1: Sample of nationally available health care databases

	Population	Payer	Health care setting	Years available	Information available
SEER	26% stratified sample of cancer patients across the United States	All payers	Inpatient/outpatient	1973–current	Diagnoses, first course of treatment, tumor site and morphology, tumor stage, patient demographics, follow-up vital status
National Surgical Quality Improvement Program of the American College of Surgeons	Surgical information from participating private-sector hospitals	All payers	Inpatient/outpatient	2001–current	Diagnoses, procedures, preoperative risk factors, intraoperative variables, mortality and morbidity outcomes
National Surgical Quality Improvement Program of the Department of Veterans Affairs	Surgical information from Veterans Affairs hospitals	Veterans Affairs only	Inpatient/outpatient	1994–current	Diagnoses, procedures, preoperative risk factors, intraoperative variables, mortality and morbidity outcomes
HCUP Nationwide Inpatient Sample	20% stratified sample of United States hospital discharges	All payers	Inpatient	1988–current	Diagnoses, procedures, discharge status, patient demographics, payment sources, total charges, lengths of stay, hospital characteristics
HCUP State Inpatient Database	Hospital discharge information from individual states	All payers	Inpatient	1990–current	Diagnoses, procedures, discharge status, patient demographics, payment sources, total charges, lengths of stay, hospital characteristics
HCUP State Ambulatory Surgery Database	Ambulatory surgery discharge information from individual states	All payers	Outpatient	1997–current	Diagnoses, procedures, patient demographics, discharge status, payment sources, total charges, hospital identifiers

HCUP Kids' Inpatient Database	National sample of hospital pediatric discharges	All payers	Inpatient	1997–current	Diagnoses, procedures, discharge status, patient demographics, payment sources, total charges, lengths of stay, hospital characteristics
HCUP State Emergency Department Databases	Emergency department encounters from participating states	All payers	Emergency department encounters	1999–current	Diagnoses, procedures, patient demographics, payment sources, total charges, hospital identifiers
Medicare Provider Analysis and Review File	Hospital discharge information	Medicare only	Inpatient	1991–2005	Diagnoses, procedures (ICD-9-CM), patient demographics, total charges, lengths of stay, vital status at discharge, follow-up vital status, entitlement data (eg, state buy-in), hospital identifiers (since 1999, fee-for-service for acute care hospitalizations only)
Medicare Hospital Outpatient Standard Analytic File	Outpatient facility services	Medicare only	Outpatient	1991–2005	Diagnoses, outpatient procedures (ICD-9-CM, HCPCS), patient demographics, charges, facility identifiers
Medicare Physician/Supplier File	Physician and other medical services	Medicare only	Inpatient and outpatient	1991–2005	Diagnoses, procedures (CPT), patient demographics, provider charges, physician identifiers

Abbreviations: CPT, Current Procedural Terminology; HCPCS, Healthcare Common Procedure Coding System; ICD-9-CM, International Classification of Diseases, 9th Revision, Clinical Modification.

[46,47]. This form of qualitative research is commonly used in business marketing. However, it can be used in hand surgery, for example, to better understand rheumatoid arthritis patients' physical limitations, physical priorities, and concerns with medical and surgical treatment options. Qualitative interviews include three main types of interviews: structured, semistructured, and in-depth. A structured interview uses a structured questionnaire; a semistructured interview uses open-ended questions; and an in-depth interview covers one or two issues in great detail with questions based on what the interviewee says [48]. Formal training in interview techniques is recommended because these interviews require considerable skill on the part of the interviewer [48]. After the qualitative research has formed the conceptual model, the questionnaire is developed. Ultimately, the questionnaire should be reliable (ie, prove the same result repeatedly in the same population under the same testing conditions), valid (ie, measure what it is supposed to measure), responsive (ie, be able to detect significant changes over time), and feasible to apply [36]. For more information on questionnaire development, we recommend reading *Health Measurement Scales: A Practical Guide to Their Development and Use* by David Streiner and Geoff Norman, Oxford Medical Publications, 2003.

Patient-reported questionnaires can be broad, general health questionnaires, or region-specific and disease-specific. Table 2 provides an alphabetical list of commonly used hand instruments. General health questionnaires, such as SF-36 [49,50] and Euroqol [51], have too wide of a focus to be useful in such specialized areas as hand surgery. However, they can be used in combination with more region- or disease-specific instruments and provide an assessment of general health status. Region-specific questionnaires include the Disabilities of the Arm and Shoulder (DASH) questionnaire [52], the American Shoulder and Elbow Surgeons questionnaire [53], the Shoulder Pain and Disability Index [54], Michigan Hand Outcomes Questionnaire (MHQ) [55], Patient Evaluation Measure (PEM) [56,57], and the Patient Related Wrist Evaluation (PRWE) [58,59]. Disease-specific questionnaires include the Australian/Canadian Osteoarthritis Hand Index [60] and the Carpal Tunnel Questionnaire (CTQ) [61]. As for measuring patient satisfaction with decisions, validated measures include the Holmes-Rovner Satisfaction with Decision Scale [62] and O'Connor's Decision Regret Scale [63].

With the multitude of hand questionnaires available today, how does a clinician choose which hand outcomes questionnaire to use? Choice of study questionnaire depends on the condition being evaluated and the conditions being studied. For example, if the study question focuses exclusively on outcomes of carpal tunnel surgery, then the CTQ [61] is the most reliable and sensitive questionnaire. However, this questionnaire has suffered from being a highly specific outcomes questionnaire used strictly for evaluation of carpal tunnel syndrome. This means that the results of this questionnaire cannot be compared to those of questionnaires for other conditions. In the United States, the DASH questionnaire and the MHQ are the most commonly used questionnaires. In the United Kingdom, the PEM is the most commonly used instrument to assess overall upper-extremity function [56]. All three are reliable and valid instruments that are very responsive to changes in patients' clinical conditions. Use of these questionnaires allows comparison amongst different conditions and patient groups. A variety of studies have compared the DASH questionnaire and MHQ with specific conditions, including carpal tunnel syndrome, and these questionnaires have been shown to be equally responsive to clinical change. We have found that the use of a general questionnaire, such as the SF-36, is too general to be applied specifically to track the outcomes of hand surgery. Table 3 provides suggestions for matching the appropriate instrument with commonly occurring hand conditions.

The PRWE has been used to evaluate hand conditions other than just wrist conditions, and this questionnaire has shown promise. There are many other types of questionnaires that have been used in the United Kingdom, such as the PEM, that may be simpler to use, have fewer questions, and impose less burden on the patient. However, with the wide variety of questionnaires that have been tested for many years and have been shown to have excellent properties, it is uncertain whether these additional questionnaires can provide any additional advantage over questionnaires currently available. The only potential advantage would be a shorter questionnaire that may have similar qualities. Patient burden is certainly a consideration when one needs to administer a variety of questionnaires to patients in addition to administering standardized hand-function testing. Minimizing patient burden should be high on the list of a researcher's considerations.

Instruments used to assess patient-reported outcomes should be reliable, valid, and responsive to change. Instrument reliability, or internal consistency, can be evaluated using the intraclass correlation coefficient (ICC) or Cronbach's alpha. The ICC, used to quantify test–retest reliability, measures the stability of responses over time when no real change is expected [64]. The ICC can range

Table 2: Patient-reported outcome instruments for hand-related conditions

Instrument	Health condition	Reliability	Validity	Responsiveness to change
Australian/Canadian Osteoarthritis Hand Index [60]	Hand osteoarthritis	ICC: 0.70 for pain; 0.77 for stiffness; 0.86 for function. CA: 0.90–0.98	r: 0.64 with global pain score; 0.72 with global function score	Decreases over time
Carpal Tunnel Questionnaire [61,85]	Assess severity of symptoms, functional status and response to treatment of the wrist and hands in patients with carpal tunnel syndrome	ICC: 0.91 for symptom severity; 0.93 for functional status	r: 0.63 with symptom severity and functional status; 0.60 with two-point discrimination and Semmes-Weinstein	Responds well to changes in patients' clinical conditions
Disabilities of the Arm and Shoulder questionnaire [85]	Upper extremity symptoms and function	ICC: 0.96	r: 0.73 with Carpal Tunnel Questionnaire; 0.72 with Shoulder Pain and Disability Index; 0.67 with pain severity at wrist	Very responsive to change and correlates well with changes in the patient's condition.
Gartland and Werley score [85]	Wrist and hand function	Unknown	Unknown	Unknown
Michigan Hand Questionnaire [55,86]	Various health states related to hand disorders, including overall hand function, activities of daily living, pain, work performance, aesthetics, patient satisfaction	ICC: 0.81 for aesthetics; 0.97 for activities of daily living. CA: 0.86 with pain scale; 0.97 with activities of daily living scale	r: 0.64 with SF-12 activities of daily living; 0.58 with SF-12 work performance; 0.79 with SF-12 pain	Responsive to patient's assessment of their clinical change
Patient Evaluation Measure [56]	Assess overall upper extremity function	CA: 0.87–0.94	r: 0.56 with pain; 0.64 with tenderness; 0.55 with swelling; −0.69 with motion; −0.76 with strength	Highly responsive (standardized response mean and effect size >1)
Patient Related Wrist Evaluation [85]	Quantify patient-reported wrist pain and disability with distal radius fractures	ICC: >0.90 for pain; >0.85 for function; >0.61 for long-term testing	r: 0.33 with SF-36 mental; 0.73 with SF-36 bodily pain; 0.52 with SF-36 functional impairment	Good
Upper Limb Functional Index [87]	Upper limb function	ICC: 0.96	r: 0.85 with Disabilities of the Arm and Shoulder questionnaire	Good

Abbreviations: CA, Cronbach's alpha; ICC, intra-class correlation; r, Pearson correlation coefficient.

from 0.00 (no agreement) to 1.00 (perfect agreement). Most agree that an ICC of 0.90 or more ensures a reliable assessment of individual patients [65]. Cronbach's alpha is used to quantify the internal consistency of items within a scale and can range from 0.00 (no correlation) to 1.00 (perfect correlation) [64]. A Cronbach's alpha of 0.8 is considered good, and a value of 0.9 is excellent

Table 3: Condition-specific instrument recommendations for patient-reported hand outcomes

Clinical condition	Instrument
Carpal tunnel syndrome	• CTQ for evaluating carpal tunnel syndrome only • DASH questionnaire and MHQ are equally valid and reliable and allow comparisons across different hand conditions
Wrist injury	• DASH questionnaire, MHQ, and PRWE are all equally valid and reliable instruments for wrist injuries
Rheumatoid arthritis	• AUSCAN for evaluating rheumatoid arthritis only • MHQ is the benchmark because it collects not only functional data but also information regarding aesthetics, symptoms, and satisfaction
Distal radius injury	• DASH questionnaire, MHQ, and PRWE are all equally valid and reliable instruments for distal radius injuries
Trauma	• DASH questionnaire and MHQ are equally valid and reliable and allow comparisons across different hand conditions

Abbreviation: AUSCAN, Australian/Canadian Osteoarthritis Hand Index.

[66]. If internal consistency is too high, such as greater than 0.9, then the scale may include too many items that are all measuring the same concept [56]. Validity is a measure of whether the items are reflecting the appropriate concept. The Pearson's correlation coefficient is often used to quantify how the instrument compares with the benchmark. Pearson's correlation coefficient ranges from $+1.0$ (perfect correlation) to -1.0 (perfect negative correlation). Finally, the instrument's ability to detect clinically important changes represents its responsiveness to change. This is measured by an effect size and by assessing the standardized response mean (SRM) [56]. Higher effect size and SRM values indicate greater responsiveness to change. An effect size of 0.2 represents a small effect, 0.5 a moderate effect, and 0.8 or greater a large effect [67].

These instruments lose validity if they are changed in any way. If modifications are deemed necessary, the instrument must undergo repeat validation testing. Investigators should resist the temptation to use in-house, nonvalidated instruments for assessing patient-reported outcomes. This practice decreases the research quality and eliminates the ability to compare the results with those from other studies [36].

A common technique to measure patient-reported outcomes is through mailed, self-administered surveys. The Dillman method [68] is a popular procedural guideline for survey administration aimed at optimizing response rates. Targeted survey response rates are 60% or higher, although the average physician survey response is 50% [69]. Poor response rates can result in a nonresponse bias and jeopardize the study's validity. Another area of bias is in the respondent's ability to recall information (ie, recall bias) [70,71]. When survey instruments obtain information subject to recall bias, statistical methods should be employed to help limit this bias. These methods include controlling for the time between the event and the survey completion and controlling for factors, such as age, that may affect an individual's ability to recall information.

Economic burden

Many different research methods can be used to evaluate economic burden of hand surgery, depending on the perspective of interest. It is important to clearly define whether the study is being made from the financial perspective of the patient, provider, society, or health care system. It is also important to assess all types of costs, including direct, indirect, and intangible costs [72].

Economic burden is an especially relevant outcome of hand surgery due to the frequency of workers' compensation claims. For example, the financial costs of a traumatic hand amputation directly affect the individual, the local health care system, the employer, and society at large from lost work productivity. Economic burden is also an important topic for managing hand trauma. Emergency departments are having difficulty finding hand surgeons to cover trauma cases because of declining reimbursement, an increase in uninsured patients, and adversarial medicolegal environments [73]. Financial analyses that address both the professional and health system operating margins can inform local and national health economic policy [74,75].

Because the United States does not have a single-payer system, most of these analyses are from single institutions [74,75]. It is difficult to combine and analyze financial data from multiple institutions. However, one statistical method that can help overcome this hurdle is the use of computer-generated predictive models, such as the Markov and Monte Carlo simulations. These computer models use computational algorithms for simulating behavior and outcomes and are especially helpful in chronic disease analyses in which patients require frequent medical and surgical care [76,77].

Cost-effective analyses are playing a more substantial role in health care policy as payers are demanding information on how much benefit is derived from each health care dollar spent. Cost utility analyses, which are a form of cost-effectiveness analyses, allow the comparison of different health outcomes by evaluating them all in terms of a single unit. This single unit is called a quality-adjusted life-year (QALY). The health units range from a 0 (death) to a 1 (perfect health). Interventions that result in a higher QALY per given dollar should be highly valued when allocating scarce health care resources [78]. Health utilities are individual's preferences for specific health states or treatments. Several methods have been used to collect data on utilities, such as the standard gamble approach, the time trade-off approach, rating scales, and the willingness-to-pay approach. These health utilities are used as preference weights within the QALY model [79,80]. Measurements of utilities help account for the indirect costs of a medical intervention, which range from loss of earnings, time to travel to the hospital, and "nonmarket" items, such as loss of lifestyle and leisure. (See the article by Thoma, Strumas, Rockwell, and McKnight in this issue.)

External funding for outcomes research in hand surgery

Several funding avenues are available to outcomes researchers in hand surgery. Investigator-funded grants can be obtained through the NIH career development awards. The NIH K23 Mentored Patient-Oriented Research Career Development Award supports clinical investigators focusing on patient-oriented research for 3 to 5 years [81]. In addition to the NIH, private foundations, such as the Robert Wood Johnson Foundation, and voluntary health organizations, such as the American Cancer Society, provide career development awards.

Project-funded grants for outcome research can be obtained through the NIH R awards. The NIH R03 is a small-grant program aimed at funding projects that can be completed within a short time with limited resources. The funding is for up to 2 years with a budget for direct costs up to $50,000 per year [82]. The NIH R21 grant is an exploratory/developmental research award. This grant is intended to support new, exploratory, and developmental research projects. Funding is for 2 years with a budget for total direct costs not to exceed $275,000 [83]. The R01 is the original and oldest grant mechanism through the NIH and can provide substantial financial support. Several private foundations, such as the Robert Wood Johnson Foundation, and medical specialty societies, such as the American Society for Surgery of the Hand, also award project grants.

The future of outcomes research in hand surgery

Hand surgery has embraced the outcomes movement. A recent audit of hand surgery outcomes studies indicates that there have been 2236 outcomes-related papers published in the Journal of Hand Surgery [83]. This audit analyzed the impact of hand surgery outcomes studies on changing the way physicians practice or on enhancing current practices. Despite enthusiastic participation in outcomes research by the hand surgery specialty, only 8% of these studies have had a level 4 impact leading to changes in current practice patterns [83]. Most of the papers have had a level 1 impact, which means they established the effectiveness of existing treatments. Surprisingly, we found only 2% of the outcomes papers were related to economic analysis projects [83]. When considering that the outcomes movement is driven by cost-containment efforts by payers to decrease variations in treatment across the United States, it is clear that investments in outcomes studies related to hand surgery have not significantly improved the quality of health care or decreased its cost. Future outcomes studies in hand surgery must challenge the current treatment paradigm by conducting more clinical trials to elevate the quality of the evidence. Hand surgery research must also consider cost within studies so that the outcomes of an intervention are considered in conjunction with economic burden on individuals and society.

The future of hand surgery outcomes research will require groups of well-trained clinical scientists capable of conducting innovative clinical research projects. The decline in clinical scientists observed over the last 20 years by the NIH still persists today, even with NIH's effort to increase funding for clinical research. An even more concerning trend is the declining number of surgeons conducting clinical trials. A strategy has been proposed in the field of plastic surgery to increase the number of clinical scientists in this specialty [84]. The recommendations call for a concerted effort to support trainees entering into established training programs funded by the NIH or the Robert Wood Johnson Foundation. A cadre of qualified surgeon clinical scientists will have the capability to engage in the 11 categories of outcomes

> Box 1: Agency for Healthcare Research and Quality categories of outcomes studies
>
> Comparative effectiveness
> Descriptive epidemiology
> Economic assessment
> Legal, legislative, or regulatory
> Methodologic development
> Modeling
> Patient-reported outcomes
> Practice variation
> Quality of health care
> Sociology of health care
> Systematic review or meta-analysis

research deemed essential by the Agency for Healthcare Research and Quality (Box 1).

By recognizing the deficiency of current hand surgery outcomes research, researchers in this specialty can start proposing ways to address these deficiencies and conduct research that can be applied in other areas. Hand surgery has a tradition of innovation and is instrumental in advancing such fields as microvascular surgery, tendon repair techniques, and implant technology. The next wave of innovation in hand surgery may involve new directions in outcomes research and clinical trials to define the most optimal treatments for our patients at affordable costs.

References

[1] Manske PR. Aesthetic hand surgery. J Hand Surg [Am] 2002;27(3):383–4.

[2] Alderman AK, Arora AS, Kuhn L, et al. An analysis of women's and men's surgical priorities and willingness to have rheumatoid hand surgery. J Hand Surg [Am] 2006;31(9):1447–53.

[3] Available at: http://www.ahrq.gov/clinic/outfact.htm. Accessed July 28, 2007.

[4] Available at: http://outcomes.cancer.gov/aboutresearch/. Accessed July 28, 2007.

[5] Weinstein JN, Bronner KK, Morgan TS, et al. Trends and geographic variations in major surgery for degenerative diseases of the hip, knee, and spine. Health Aff (Millwood) 2004;(Suppl Web Exclusives):VAR81–9.

[6] Baicker K, Chandra A, Skinner JS, et al. Who you are and where you live: how race and geography affect the treatment of Medicare beneficiaries. Health Aff (Millwood) 2004;(Suppl Web Exclusives):VAR33–44.

[7] Skinner J, Weinstein JN, Sporer SM, et al. Racial, ethnic, and geographic disparities in rates of knee arthroplasty among Medicare patients. N Engl J Med 2003;349(14):1350–9.

[8] Milner PC, Payne JN, Stanfield RC, et al. Inequalities in accessing hip joint replacement for people in need. Eur J Public Health 2004;14(1):58–62.

[9] Beckmann K, Iosifidis P, Shorne L, et al. Effects of variations in hysterectomy status on population coverage by cervical screening. Aust N Z J Public Health 2003;27(5):507–12.

[10] Available at: http://www.ahrq.gov/about/whatis.htm. Accessed August 2, 2007.

[11] Alderman AK, Wei Y, Birkmeyer JD. Use of breast reconstruction after mastectomy following the Women's Health and Cancer Rights Act. JAMA 2006;295(4):387–8.

[12] Alderman AK, McMahon L, Wilkins EG. The national utilization of immediate and early delayed breast reconstruction & the impact of sociodemographic factors. Plastic and Reconstructive Surgery 2003;11:695–703.

[13] Alderman AK, Kim HM, Kotsis SV, et al. Upper-extremity sarcomas in the United States: analysis of the surveillance, epidemiology, and end results database, 1973–1998. J Hand Surg [Am] 2003;28(3):511–8.

[14] Chung KC, Kowalski CP, Walters MR. Finger replantation in the United States: rates and resource use from the 1996 Healthcare Cost and Utilization Project. J Hand Surg [Am] 2000;25(6):1038–42.

[15] Alderman AK, Chung KC, Demonner S, et al. The rheumatoid hand: a predictable disease with unpredictable surgical practice patterns. Arthritis Rheum 2002;47(5):537–42.

[16] Alderman AK, Chung KC, Kim HM, et al. Effectiveness of rheumatoid hand surgery: contrasting perceptions of hand surgeons and rheumatologists. J Hand Surg [Am] 2003;28(1):3–11 [discussion: 12–3].

[17] Alderman AK, Ubel PA, Kim HM, et al. Surgical management of the rheumatoid hand: consensus and controversy among rheumatologists and hand surgeons. J Rheumatol 2003;30(7):1464–72.

[18] Available at: https://acsnsqip.org/login/default.aspx. Accessed July 29, 2007.

[19] Available at: http://www.ahrq.gov/data/hcup/. Accessed July 29, 2007.

[20] Cooper GS, Yuan Z, Stange KC, et al. Agreement of Medicare claims and tumor registry data for assessment of cancer-related treatment. Med Care 2000;38(4):411–21.

[21] Chung KC, Kotsis SV, Kim HM. A prospective outcomes study of Swanson metacarpophalangeal joint arthroplasty for the rheumatoid hand. J Hand Surg Am 2004;29(4):646–53.

[22] Nakagawa N, Abe S, Saegusa Y, et al. Long-term results of open elbow synovectomy for rheumatoid arthritis. Modern Rheumatology 2007;17(2):106–9.

[23] Stanley K. Evaluation of randomized controlled trials. Circulation 2007;115(13):1819–22.

[24] Chung KC, Kalliainen LK, Spilson SV, et al. The prevalence of negative studies with inadequate statistical power: an analysis of the plastic surgery literature. Plastic & Reconstructive Surgery 2002;109(1):1–6 [discussion: 7–8].

[25] Chung KC, Kalliainen LK, Hayward RA. Type II (beta) errors in the hand literature: the importance of power. J Hand Surg [Am] 1998;23(1): 20–5.

[26] Chung KC, Burns PB, Kim HM. A practical guide to meta-analysis. J Hand Surg [Am] 2006;31(10): 1671–8.

[27] Available at: http://en.wikipedia.org/wiki/Meta-analysis. Accessed July 28, 2007.

[28] Chung KC, Kowalski CP, Myra Kim H, et al. Patient outcomes following Swanson silastic metacarpophalangeal joint arthroplasty in the rheumatoid hand: a systematic overview. J Rheumatol 2000;27(6):1395–402.

[29] Available at: http://en.wikipedia.org/wiki/Systematic_review. Accessed July 28, 2007.

[30] Kotsis SV, Chung KC. A systematic review of the outcomes of digital sympathectomy for treatment of chronic digital ischemia. J Rheumatol 2003;30(8):1788–92.

[31] Needleman IG. A guide to systematic reviews. J Clin Periodontol 2002;(29 Suppl 3):6–9 [discussion: 37–8].

[32] Thoma A, Veltri K, Haines T, et al. A systematic review of reviews comparing the effectiveness of endoscopic and open carpal tunnel decompression. Plast Reconstr Surg 2004;113(4):1184–91.

[33] Martou G, Veltri K, Thoma A. Surgical treatment of osteoarthritis of the carpometacarpal joint of the thumb: a systematic review. Plast Reconstr Surg 2004;114(2):421–32.

[34] Available at: http://en.wikipedia.org/wiki/Cochrane_Collaboration. Accessed July 28, 2007.

[35] Kotsis SV, Lau FH, Chung KC. Responsiveness of the Michigan Hand Outcomes Questionnaire and physical measurements in outcome studies of distal radius fracture treatment. J Hand Surg [Am] 2007;32(1):84–90.

[36] Bindra RR, Dias JJ, Heras-Palau C, et al. Assessing outcome after hand surgery: the current state. J Hand Surg [Br] 2003;28(4):289–94.

[37] Bradley MP, Hayes EP, Weiss AP, et al. A prospective study of outcome following mini-open carpal tunnel release. Hand Surg 2003;8(1):59–63.

[38] Chung KC, Kotsis SV, Kim HM. Predictors of functional outcomes after surgical treatment of distal radius fractures. J Hand Surg [Am] 2007; 32(1):76–83.

[39] LaStayo PC, Wheeler DL. Reliability of passive wrist flexion and extension goniometric measurements: a multicenter study. Phys Ther 1994;74(2):162–74 [discussion: 174–6].

[40] Atroshi I, Larsson GU, Ornstein E, et al. Outcomes of endoscopic surgery compared with open surgery for carpal tunnel syndrome among employed patients: randomised controlled trial. BMJ 2006;332(7556):1473.

[41] Rab M, Grunbeck M, Beck H, et al. Intra-individual comparison between open and 2-portal endoscopic release in clinically matched bilateral carpal syndrome. J Plast Reconstr Aesthet Surg 2006;59(7):730–6.

[42] Available at: http://www.nihpromis.org/default.aspx. Accessed August 5, 2007.

[43] Available at: http://nihroadmap.nih.gov/clinicalresearch/promis.asp. Accessed August 5, 2007.

[44] Meadows KA. So you want to do research? 5: Questionnaire design. Br J Community Nurs 2003;8(12):562–70.

[45] Rattray J, Jones MC. Essential elements of questionnaire design and development. J Clin Nurs 2007;16(2):234–43.

[46] Parsons M, Greenwood J. A guide to the use of focus groups in health care research: Part 1. Contemp Nurse 2000;9(2):169–80.

[47] Webb B. Using focus groups as a research method: a personal experience. J Nurs Manag 2002;10(1):27–35.

[48] Britten N. Qualitative interviews in medical research. Bmj 1995;311(6999):251–3.

[49] Ware JE Jr, Sherbourne CD. The MOS 36-Item Short-Form Health Survey (SF-36). I. Conceptual framework and item selection. Med Care 1992; 30(6):473–83.

[50] Ware JE Jr. Patient-based assessment: tools for monitoring and improving healthcare outcomes. Behav Healthc Tomorrow 1996;5(3):88.

[51] EuroQol—a new facility for the measurement of health-related quality of life. The EuroQol Group. Health Policy 1990;16(3):199–208.

[52] Hudak PL, Amadio PC, Bombardier C. Development of an upper extremity outcome measure: the DASH (disabilities of the arm, shoulder and hand) [corrected]. The Upper Extremity Collaborative Group (UECG). Am J Ind Med 1996; 29(6):602–8.

[53] Richards R, An KN, Bigliani LU, et al. American shoulder and elbow surgeons. A standardized method for the assessment of the shoulder function. J Shoulder Elbow Surg 1994;3: 347–52.

[54] Roach KE, Budiman-Mak E, Songsiridej N, et al. Development of a shoulder pain and disability index. Arthritis Care Res 1991;4(4):143–9.

[55] Chung KC, Pillsbury MS, Walters MR, et al. Reliability and validity testing of the Michigan Hand Outcomes Questionnaire. J Hand Surg [Am] 1998;23(4):575–87.

[56] Dias JJ, Bhowal B, Wildin CJ, et al. Assessing the outcome of disorders of the hand. Is the patient evaluation measure reliable, valid, responsive and without bias? J Bone Joint Surg Br 2001; 83(2):235–40.

[57] Hobby JL, Watts C, Elliot D. Validity and responsiveness of the patient evaluation measure as an outcome measure for carpal tunnel syndrome. J Hand Surg [Br] 2005;30(4):350–4.

[58] MacDermid JC, Turgeon T, Richards RS, et al. Patient rating of wrist pain and disability: a reliable and valid measurement tool. J Orthop Trauma 1998;12(8):577–86.

[59] MacDermid JC, Richards RS, Donner A, et al. Responsiveness of the Short Form-36, Disability of the Arm, Shoulder, and Hand questionnaire,

[59] Patient-Rated Wrist evaluation, and Physical Impairment Measurements in evaluating recovery after a distal radius fracture. J Hand Surg [Am] 2000;25(2):330–40.
[60] Bellamy N, Campbell J, Haraoui B, et al. Clinimetric properties of the AUSCAN Osteoarthritis Hand Index: an evaluation of reliability, validity and responsiveness. Osteoarthritis & Cartilage 2002;10(11):863–9.
[61] Levine DW, Simmons BP, Koris MJ, et al. A self-administered questionnaire for the assessment of severity of symptoms and functional status in carpal tunnel syndrome. J Bone Joint Surg Am 1993;75(11):1585–92.
[62] Holmes-Rovner M, Kroll J, Schmitt N, et al. Patient satisfaction with health care decisions: the satisfaction with decision scale. Med Decis Making 1996;16(1):58–64.
[63] Brehaut JC, O'Connor AM, Wood TJ, et al. Validation of a decision regret scale. Med Decis Making 2003;23(4):281–92.
[64] Angst F, Goldhahn J, Pap G, et al. Cross-cultural adaptation, reliability and validity of the German Shoulder Pain and Disability Index (SPADI). Rheumatology (Oxford) 2007;46(1):87–92.
[65] Bot SD, Terwee CB, van der Windt DA, et al. Clinimetric evaluation of shoulder disability questionnaires: a systematic review of the literature. Ann Rheum Dis 2004;63(4):335–41.
[66] Feinstein A. Clinimetrics. New Haven (CT): Yale University Press; 1987. p. 180.
[67] Cohen J. Applied multiple regression/correlation analysis for the behavioral sciences. Hillsdale (NJ): Lawrence Erlbaum Associates; 1983.
[68] Anema MG, Brown BE. Increasing survey responses using the total design method. J Contin Educ Nurs 1995;26(3):109–14.
[69] Cummings SM, Savitz LA, Konrad TR. Reported response rates to mailed physician questionnaires. Health Serv Res 2001;35(6):1347–55.
[70] Houtveen JH, Oei NY. Recall bias in reporting medically unexplained symptoms comes from semantic memory. J Psychosom Res 2007;62(3):277–82.
[71] Barry D, Livingstone V. The investigation and correction of recall bias for an ordinal response in a case-control study. Stat Med 2006;25(6):965–75.
[72] Pizzi L, Lofland JH, Elwood C, editors. Economic evaluation in U.S. health care: principles and applications. Sudbury (MA): Jones and Bartlett; 2005. p. 2–9.
[73] Burt CW, McCaig LF. Staffing, capacity, and ambulance diversion in emergency departments: United States, 2003–04. Adv Data 2006;(376):1–23.
[74] Alderman AK, Storey A, Chung KC. Financial impact of emergency hand trauma on the healthcare system. J Am Coll Surg, in press.
[75] Hasan JS, Chung KC, Storey AF, et al. Financial impact of hand surgery programs on academic medical centers. Plast Reconstr Surg 2007;119(2):627–35.
[76] Bell C, Graham J, Earnshaw S, et al. Cost-effectiveness of four immunomodulatory therapies for relapsing-remitting multiple sclerosis: a Markov model based on long-term clinical data. J Manag Care Pharm 2007;13(3):245–61.
[77] Anderson K, Jacobson JS, Heitjan DF, et al. Cost-effectiveness of preventive strategies for women with a BRCA1 or a BRCA2 mutation. Ann Intern Med 2006;144(6):397–406.
[78] McGregor M. Cost-utility analysis: Use QALYs only with great caution. CMAJ 2003;68(4):433–4.
[79] Available at: www.evidence-based-medicine.co.uk. Accessed July 28, 2007.
[80] Available at: http://www.jr2.ox.ac.uk/bandolier/painres/download/whatis/Health-util.pdf. Accessed July 28, 2007.
[81] Available at: http://grants2.nih.gov/grants/guide/pa-files/PA-00-004.html. Accessed August 1, 2007.
[82] Available at: http://grants.nih.gov/grants/funding/r03.htm. Accessed August 1, 2007.
[83] Chung KC, Burns PB, Davis Sears E. Outcomes research in hand surgery: Where have we been and where should we go? J Hand Surg [Am] 2006;31(8):1373–9.
[84] Chung K. Revitalizing the training of the clinical scientists in surgery. Plast Reconstr Surg, in press.
[85] Changulani M, Okonkwo U, Keswani T, et al. Outcome evaluation measures for wrist and hand—which one to choose? Int Orthop 2007 May 30; [Epub ahead of print].
[86] Chung KC, Hamill JB, Walters MR, et al. The Michigan Hand Outcomes Questionnaire (MHQ): assessment of responsiveness to clinical change. Ann Plast Surg 1999;42(6):619–22.
[87] Gabel CP, Michener LA, Burkett B, et al. The Upper Limb Functional Index: development and determination of reliability, validity, and responsiveness. J Hand Ther 2006;19(3):328–48, quiz 349.

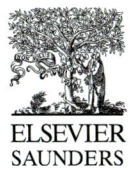

Clinical Research in Pediatric Plastic Surgery and Systematic Review of Quality-of-Life Questionnaires

Anne F. Klassen, DPhil[a],*, Mitchell A. Stotland, MD[b], Erik D. Skarsgard, MD[c], Andrea L. Pusic, MD, MHS[d]

- Study designs used in pediatric plastic surgery research
  Case series
  Case-control studies
  Cohort studies
  Randomized controlled trials
  Systematic reviews
- Measurement of outcome in pediatric plastic surgery
  Traditional outcome measures
  Quality-of-life outcomes

  Systematic review of quality-of-life instruments in pediatric plastic surgery
- Methodology
- Results
  Burns
  Craniofacial
  Pectus excavatum
- Discussion
- Summary
- Acknowledgments
- References

Study designs used in pediatric plastic surgery research

The practice of evidence-based medicine requires the availability of high-quality clinical trials within the scientific literature and an ability to discern levels of research evidence. The hierarchy of evidence in clinical reporting is generally understood to ascend in the following sequence: expert opinion, case report/series, case-control study, cohort study, randomized controlled trial (RCT), meta-analysis, and systematic review (see the article by Sprague, McKay, and Thoma in this issue). Designing an exemplary clinical study in pediatric plastic surgery is complicated by the fact that many of the desired outcomes (eg, symmetry, contour, aesthetic balance and harmony, volume, three-dimensional position, vocal quality) are difficult to measure objectively. Moreover, many clinical conditions within the scope of pediatric plastic surgical care are uncommon, making accrual of a large series of patients a challenge. These factors help to

---

[a] Department of Pediatrics, McMaster University, IAHS Building, Room 408D, 1400 Main Street West, Hamilton, ON L8S 1C7, Canada
[b] Craniofacial Anomalies Clinic, Dartmouth-Hitchcock Medical Center, One Medical Center Drive, Lebanon, NH 03755, USA
[c] Department of Surgery (Pediatric General Surgery), University of British Columbia, KO-123 ACB 4480 Oak Street, Vancouver, BC V6H 3V4, Canada
[d] Plastic and Reconstructive Surgery, Memorial Sloan-Kettering Cancer Center, 1275 York Avenue, New York, NY 10021, USA
* Corresponding author.
E-mail address: aklass@mcmaster.ca (A.F. Klassen).

explain to why evolution in the quality of clinical reporting in pediatric plastic surgery has occurred at a slower pace than in many other areas of medicine.

Case series

Case series, despite ranking low in quality of evidence, may impart indispensable management pearls that greatly advance clinical care. The most valuable case series are usually technique-oriented articles produced by pediatric plastic surgeons with a large practical experience, describe clever procedural innovations that make intuitive sense, address existing treatment challenges, exhibit convincing clinical photographs (although typically nonrandomly selected), and present novel concepts in a cogent manner. Classic examples of important case series in pediatric plastic surgery include those on cleft lip repair by Millard [1] and by Mulliken [2]; on cleft palate repair by Furlow [3]; on craniofacial surgery by Tessier [4] and by Kawamoto [5]; and on microtia reconstruction by Tanzer [6], Brent [7], and Nagata [8]. Without measurable outcomes available, however, the ability of one to appreciate the merit of a new treatment innovation described within a case series requires some intuition and the perspective of time and experience.

Case-control studies

Case-control studies are observational in nature. They identify individuals with and without a particular condition of interest ("cases" and "controls") and then look retrospectively to find predictor variables that may explain why patients developed their condition. This type of epidemiologic research has not been characteristic of the pediatric plastic surgery literature, which focuses more closely on the effects of surgical intervention. Case-control studies investigating clinical disorders of plastic surgical interest do exist, however, and include reports examining maternal cigarette smoking and craniosynostosis [9]; the neurodevelopment of infants with craniosynostosis [10]; the effect of maternal alcohol [11], stress [12], and folic acid intake [13] on orofacial clefting; and the influence of cigarette use on the development of clefts [14] and digital anomalies [15]. These types of studies are important in helping to understand the cause of rare conditions. Their major shortcomings are that they do not lend themselves readily to evaluating plastic surgical interventions and that, by being retrospective in nature, they are highly susceptible to bias.

Cohort studies

As opposed to case series, cohort studies follow a group of subjects over time and measure predictor variables and outcomes in a more rigorous manner. Cohort studies play a major role in advancing knowledge in pediatric plastic surgery because of the difficulty in implementing RCTs to test new surgical interventions. The contributors of case series often go on to assemble important retrospective cohort studies to establish the value of their original work and ideas convincingly. Examples include the systematic clinical surveillance demonstrated in articles by McComb and Coghlan [16] on the cleft nasal deformity, by Berkowitz and colleagues [17] on cleft dentoskeletal growth, by Shetye and colleagues [18] on mandibular distraction osteogenesis, by Brent [19] on microtia, and by McCarthy and colleagues [20] and by Becker and colleagues [21] on craniosynostosis. The strength of evidence of cohort studies depends on the completeness of follow-up of subjects and the accuracy of measurement, which ultimately determine the quality of the data. The conclusions of even the most thorough and comprehensive cohort studies need to be interpreted with the understanding that many of the outcome variables in pediatric plastic surgery are entirely subjective in nature.

Randomized controlled trials

An RCT represents a true experiment. An intervention is performed, and outcomes are prospectively measured, comparing randomly selected treatment and control groups (see the article by Thoma, Sprague, Temple, and Archibald in this issue).

There is a paucity of RCTs in pediatric plastic surgery. This may be explained by a variety of reasons. Alternative surgical treatments tend to evolve gradually over time rather than in quantum steps. Clearly, distinct treatment options may not necessarily exist. Collection of adequate sample size for statistical analysis is difficult when considering relatively rare congenital anomalies. Individual surgeons may not have equivalent expertise in alternative interventions (eg, autologous versus alloplastic reconstruction for microtia, open versus endoscopic approach to sagittal craniosynostosis). Sometimes, when appealing quantum leaps have occurred, they have been embraced so rapidly that it would be unlikely for a clinician to be willing to compare the new technique randomly with the old (eg, distraction osteogenesis versus standard osteotomy for LeFort III advancement). One notable effort to use a multi-institutional randomized controlled study design for oral clefts has emerged from the Netherlands. The Dutchcleft team involved treatment centers in Amsterdam, Nijmegen, and Rotterdam. This study group has used an RCT to examine the effect of infant orthopedics carefully on a variety of important outcome measures in children with cleft lip/palate [22].

This group used an RCT to examine the effect of infant orthopedics on a variety of important outcome measures in children with unilateral cleft lip and palate. New study subjects were enrolled over a 4-year period and were randomized into treatment (passive infant orthopedic device applied within 2 weeks of birth and worn until palate repair at 52 weeks of age) and control (no orthopedic device) groups. A series of detailed articles describe their findings, which indicate that passive infant orthopedic devices for unilateral cleft lip and palate do not provide significant benefit in terms of maxillary arch dimensions, alveolar segment collapse, deciduous dental occlusion, or feeding and nutritional status [22–25].

Another multi-institutional group has recently used an RCT to compare the effect of pharyngeal flap versus sphincteroplasty surgery for the treatment of velopharyngeal insufficiency. Using a rigorous study methodology, the Velopharyngeal Insufficiency Surgical Trial Group was unable to demonstrate a significant difference between the two interventions in terms of efficacy or safety [26]. Limitations of both of these studies include the ultimate subjectivity of some of the outcome measures (eg, perceptual speech, endoscopic assessment of velopharyngeal closure) and the difficulty in controlling for variability in technique between different surgeons. Senders and colleagues [27] performed a single-center, placebo-controlled, double-blind RCT looking at the effect of perioperative steroids in cleft palate repair. The evidence of the study was constrained by a small sample size (N = 45) that included six different surgical techniques, no mention of the number of surgeons participating, and the subjectivity of the outcome measure "airway distress." Fearon and Weinthal [28] used an RCT to examine the use of preoperative erythropoietin in reducing transfusion requirements in a pediatric population undergoing craniosynostosis repair. This study involved a single surgeon, all evaluators were blinded to treatment, and strict criteria were used for transfusion. The method of randomization was not described, however, and the two study groups were not statistically compared in terms of age, weight, and diagnosis. Gross inspection of the two groups indicates that there was a greater requirement for fronto-orbital osteotomy and advancement in the control group; thus, it is questionable how similar the surgical procedures were in the two groups.

Systematic reviews

There are few examples of meta-analyses and systematic reviews pertaining to pediatric plastic surgical conditions. These types of composite reports may yield the highest level of clinic evidence only if they can incorporate multiple high-quality studies for consideration (see the article by Haines, McKnight, Duku, Perry, and Thoma in this issue). Glenny and colleagues [29] performed a systematic review investigating alternative feeding interventions for growth and development in infants with facial clefts. Their main criterion for inclusion was RCTs examining infants up to 6 months of age with cleft lip or palate. Subjects were considered before and after surgery for cleft repair. The feeding interventions considered comprised a wide variety of techniques, including squeezable versus rigid bottles, maxillary plate versus no maxillary plate, and breastfeeding versus spoon-feeding. Only 4 studies were identified, with a total of 232 babies. From a clinical perspective, this systematic review was unable to provide meaningful information because of the marked heterogeneity in subject age, diagnosis, and clinical stage and in the diversity of treatments considered.

Liao and Mars [30] published a systematic review examining the association between timing of hard palatal cleft repair and later facial growth. They searched the English literature over the preceding 38-year period for the keywords "facial growth," "cleft lip palate," and "timing of (hard) palate repair." Fifteen retrospective nonrandomized studies were considered. The studies were found to be markedly heterogeneous in terms of timing of hard palate repair and outcome parameters measured. Methodologic deficiencies were widespread and categorized as inappropriate sampling, inadequate assessment, inappropriate statistics, and inadequate duration of follow-up. No meta-analysis could be performed because of the diversity of studies, and no major conclusions could be made from the review.

Finally, Bialocerkowski and colleagues [31] performed a high-quality systematic review, searching 13 databases for quantitative studies on the effectiveness of conservative treatment for positional plagiocephaly. The search was limited to the English literature over the preceding 20-year period. Sixteen papers were included in the review, and all were critically appraised using previously established methods. The methodologic quality of the studies was deemed moderate to poor, however. Little detail was revealed regarding actual treatment undertaken, subject age, type of physical therapy, and method of fabrication of orthotic helmets. There was a wide variation in outcome measures used and little mention of accuracy and reliability of anthropomorphic measures that were used. None of the studies used a randomization protocol. Therefore, clinically significant conclusions were unable to be drawn from this systematic review.

Measurement of outcome in pediatric plastic surgery

Traditional outcome measures

In addition to choosing a study design to answer a clinical question, another important decision concerns the particular outcome measures to include in the study. The pediatric plastic surgery literature has many examples of clinical studies in which the focus of assessment has been on traditional measures of outcome, such as complication rates, measures of morbidity and aesthetic concerns. For example, studies of distraction osteogenesis for craniofacial anomalies have focused on cephalometric analysis and review of complications [32–34], studies of vascular malformation have examined radiographic outcomes [35,36], and the cleft lip and palate literature has considered facial measurements and photographs [37,38]. Although traditional measures of outcome are important, they do not capture the full range of ways in which a child may be affected by his or her condition. Broader measures of outcome, such as child and family perceptions of quality of life (QOL), have been less well examined, but researchers have become increasingly cognizant that it is the patient's perception of the outcome that ultimately determines the success of a procedure.

Quality-of-life outcomes

To measure a broader range of outcomes in pediatric plastic surgery, a growing number of multidimensional "quality-of-life" or "health-related quality-of-life" (both referred to herewith as QOL) questionnaires have been developed and can be used to assess the impact of plastic surgery on the health and well-being of children. QOL questionnaires are based on the view that health is multidimensional, that the concepts forming these dimensions can be assessed only by subjective measures, and that QOL should be evaluated by asking the patient or, in some cases, a proxy. Pediatric QOL assessment has come to be recognized as an important health outcome in children, and research in this area has grown substantially since 1980, as evident in Fig. 1. For pediatric plastic surgery researchers who seek to report these outcomes accurately, a thorough understanding of the issues specific to pediatric QOL measurement is essential.

The category of QOL instruments that are applicable to many patients, regardless of their health condition, are called generic instruments. Generic questionnaires allow direct comparisons across disease groups or between sick and healthy groups. Their disadvantage is that they sometimes lack sensitivity to the particular concerns of a patient group.

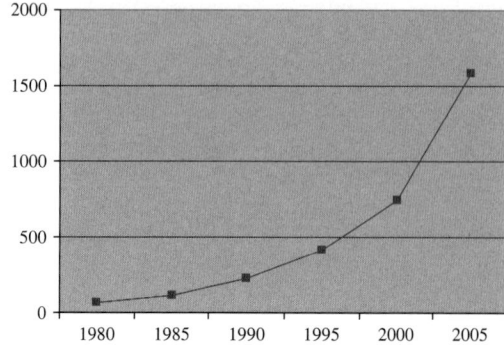

Fig. 1. Number of articles using the phrase "quality of life" and limited to children aged 0 to 18 years as identified in the PubMed database (1980–2005).

Disease- or condition-specific instruments, conversely, address problems specific to only one illness or disease. Such instruments, when developed through in-depth qualitative interviews with children, can help to identify QOL issues of importance to them. Although they are likely to be sensitive to small changes in health, however, they cannot be used to compare across particular patient groups. A comprehensive approach involves supplementing generic instruments with condition- or disease-specific instruments to capture information on the major domains common to all diseases and to the ones unique to the particular condition of interest [39]. To facilitate this approach, some generic QOL instruments have disease-specific modules, but there are also many disease-specific modules that have been developed independently.

In choosing an instrument for a pediatric plastic surgery study, in addition to considering the psychometric properties of the instrument (eg, reliability, validity, responsiveness), one needs to be clear about which domains are of most relevance to the research questions being asked. The content and psychometric properties of a range of generic and condition- or disease-specific QOL instruments developed for children and adolescents have been extensively reviewed [40–53]. Most recently, Davis and colleagues [51] identified 14 generic and 25 condition-specific QOL instruments developed for children aged 0 to 12 years. The aim of that article was to appraise critically the conceptual frameworks of QOL instruments. These investigators report that QOL was assessed by a variety of domains, including emotional, social, and physical health and well-being. In the same year, Ravens-Sieberer and colleagues [52] published a review of generic and disease-specific QOL instruments developed for children aged 2 to 18 years. MEDLINE and PsycINFO were searched between 1980 and 2006, and more than 50 QOL instruments were identified. Among the conclusions, these investigators highlight that generic QOL instruments are available to assess domains important to children and adolescents, and they recommend 10 conceptually and scientifically sound instruments. Of the 5 generic instruments used in studies that involved patients with conditions treated by plastic surgeons (Table 1), 6 of these instruments are ones recommended by Ravens-Sieberer and colleagues [52]. Other conclusions by this team were that QOL of children and adolescents can and should be ascertained using self-report and that measurement instruments used to assess QOL need to consider maturity and cognitive development. These findings raise important issues particular to measuring QOL in pediatric populations, which are examined in more detail here.

Self- and proxy report of quality of life

The premise underlying QOL assessment is that the individual is the best observer and reporter of his or

Table 1: Generic pediatric QOL instruments used in studies of children with conditions treated by plastic surgeons

Measure	Domains covered	Pediatric plastic surgery study in which measure used
Child health and illness profile [54][a]	Achievement, discomfort, disorders, resilience, risks, satisfaction	Oral clefts [55]
Child health questionnaire [56][a]	Physical functioning, physical role/social functioning, general health perceptions, bodily pain/discomfort, general behavior, mental health, self-esteem, emotional role/social functioning, change in health, parental impact (emotional), parental impact (time), family activities, family cohesion	Craniofacial [57], burns [58,59,60]
Infant and toddler quality of life [61,62]	Physical abilities, growth and development, pain/discomfort, temperament and moods, general behavior, getting along with others, general health perception, change in health, parental impact (emotional), parental impact (time), parental mental health, parental general health perception, family cohesion	Burns [63]
KINDL [64][a]	Psychologic well-being, social relationships, physical functioning, everyday life activities	Cleft lip and palate [65]
Pediatric Quality of Life Inventory [66][a]	Physical, social, emotional and school function	[67]
TNO-AZL Child Quality of Life Questionnaire [68][a]	Pain and symptoms, social functioning, motor functioning, autonomy, cognitive functioning, negative global emotional functioning, positive global emotional functioning	Neurofibromatosis type 1 [69], sagittal craniosynostosis [70], burns [71]
Youth quality of life instrument [72][a]	Self, relationships, environment, general quality of life	Facial differences [73,74]

[a] Conceptually and scientifically sound generic measures of pediatric QOL according to Ravens-Sieberer and colleagues [52].

her own health. Patient self-report is indeed considered the standard in patient-reported outcomes measurement [75,76]. For children, however, this method is not always feasible or possible for health conditions in which the child may be too ill to complete questionnaires by himself or herself; unwilling to do so; or lacking the necessary language skills, attention, or cognitive abilities. Proxies (usually the parent) may need to provide information on the child's behalf. Moreover, even when children are able to participate, proxy ratings may provide a different perspective that is complementary. The validity of proxy report is thus an important topic and has been the subject of a growing number of studies. Eiser and Morse [43] reviewed 14 studies that assessed the relation between parent-proxy and child self-reported QOL and demonstrated that agreement between parents and children seemed to depend on the domain. Agreement was generally good for more observable domains of QOL, such as physical function and behavior, and was generally poor for less observable domains, such as social or emotional function/well-being.

Recently, a few studies have used qualitative techniques to understand parent-child differences better in reporting of child QOL, although more research of this nature is needed. Davis and colleagues [77] used the think-aloud technique to study the thought processes behind how parents and children answer a QOL questionnaire and found that parents and children tend to base their answers on different experiences or use different response styles. Ungar and colleagues [78] took a different approach and administered a range of validated QOL instruments to a small sample of children with asthma in Ontario to observe and describe the interaction between parent and child and to identify strategies parents use to enable their child to answer questionnaire items as accurately as possible. Parents were found to be a valuable resource in overcoming problems associated with inaccurate recall, respondent bias, frustration, discomfort, anxiety, and comprehension.

Developmental considerations

Given that parent and child report of child QOL differ, particularly for domains that are not observable, it is important to collect self-report data whenever possible. Although a young child may not have the cognitive abilities needed to complete a QOL measure, older children, and especially adolescents, are able to self-report on their health accurately and reliably. This was shown by Riley [79], who reviewed several different bodies of research, including cognitive development, psychometric studies, cognitive interviewing research, and longitudinal research, and found that children can successfully complete age-appropriate health questionnaires. Her review provided evidence to show that children as young as 6 years of age are able to understand questions about their QOL and to give valid and reliable answers. Other research has shown that children as young as 3 or 4 years old can self-report on pain and nausea [80].

As the value of obtaining child self-report of QOL is increasingly recognized, there is still much research needed to determine the best ways to measure QOL in children. To ensure that self-report data are valid and reliable, the development of pediatric QOL questionnaires must consider the age, maturity, and emotional and cognitive development of the target audience and how these characteristics change over time [79]. It is also important to measure dimensions of QOL that are important and relevant to the particular patient group of interest.

Developing a quality-of-life instrument

There are numerous ways in which pediatric QOL instruments can vary (eg, recall period, length, mode of administration, format, content). This was pointed out by Cremeens and colleagues [50], who recently reviewed 53 health-related self-report instruments for children aged 3 to 8 years of age to find out more about different techniques and formats used. These investigators described a range of response scales and presentation styles that have been used to date and call for the development of a set of minimum standards for child self-report instruments and for further research to reach a consensus as to the most appropriate format for child self-report instruments.

QOL instruments need to be properly developed using appropriate methods to ensure that they are scientifically sound and clinically meaningful. To develop a QOL measure for children, the authors recommend following the three-stage method summarized by Cano and colleagues [81], which is based on guidelines set by the Scientific Advisory Committee of the Medical Outcomes Trust [82]. The first step involves defining the conceptual model to be measured and generating a pool of items to ensure that all important areas are considered for inclusion in the final scale. Preliminary versions of the instrument are then developed from three sources: review of the literature, qualitative interviews with patients (this must involve children), and expert opinion. The item pool is then pretested or piloted on a small sample of patients to clarify ambiguities in the wording of items, confirm appropriateness, and determine acceptability and completion time. In the second step, field testing is performed on a larger sample of patients. Questions are eliminated according to item redundancy, endorsement frequencies, missing data, factor analysis, and tests of scaling assumptions. This "item-reduction" process completes the instrument development. In the final step, psychometric evaluation or validation of the measure is performed; the instrument, in its final form, is administered to a large population of patients to determine questionnaire acceptability, internal consistency reliability, item total correlations, test-retest reliability, validity within scale, validity in comparison with other instruments, and responsiveness.

Systematic review of quality-of-life instruments in pediatric plastic surgery

The authors conducted a systematic literature review to identify and appraise condition-specific instruments developed for use by children with conditions treated by plastic surgeons. Such a review is needed to identify and focus future research efforts toward areas in which there are currently no instruments available.

Methodology

MEDLINE, Cinahl, EMBASE, PsycINFO, and Sociological Abstracts were searched from the inception of each database to May 2007. MEDLINE search terms included (and were modified for the other databases) "quality of life," "health status," "well-being," and "patient-reported outcome." These were combined with search terms for plastic, reconstructive, aesthetic, or cosmetic surgery and a list of 99 terms covering specific plastic surgery procedures and conditions treated by plastic surgeons. The search was limited to children aged 0 to 18 years, but no limitation was made on language. Articles were included if they described a condition-specific QOL measure developed specifically for use with children, and the study included children with conditions treated by plastic surgeons. Articles that focused exclusively on specific aspects of well-being, (eg, pain, self-esteem) were excluded because they did not assess overall QOL. Articles that described instruments that did not provide evidence of any development or validation process (ie, ad hoc instruments) were excluded, as were articles that described instruments developed for adults but used in studies that involved children.

The titles and abstracts of each article were examined by two reviewers, and the full text of all potentially relevant papers was obtained and examined, also by two reviewers. If an examined paper contained no information regarding instrument development or validation, the corresponding author was contacted by e-mail and asked if there was an article describing the instrument's development and validation. The references of each article included in the review were examined to identify additional articles that met the search criteria.

Information from each article meeting study inclusion criteria was extracted by two reviewers. Articles that described a condition-specific QOL questionnaire were appraised for adherence to "gold standard" guidelines for health outcomes instrument development, as summarized by Cano and colleagues [81] and described previously.

Results

A total of 945 articles were identified by the authors' search strategy, of which 63 articles were examined in detail and 11 were found to meet the inclusion criteria [58,59,63,83–90]. A secondary search of the reference lists from these articles and other articles found by the authors added 12 additional articles [74,91–101], resulting in a total of 23 studies that used eight condition-specific instruments. Questionnaires have been developed to measure QOL in the following three areas: burns (n = 1), craniofacial anomalies (n = 6), and pectus excavatum (n = 1). Table 2 summarizes information pertaining to the domains of reliability, validity, and responsiveness of each instrument.

Burns

The American Burn Association/Shriners Hospitals for Children Burn Outcomes Questionnaire (BOQ) was developed to measure QOL issues in children with burns. A 55-item parent form is available for measuring QOL in children aged 0 to 5 years [87]. For children between the ages of 5 and 18 years, a separate 52-item form is available for parent completion, and there is a version for adolescents aged 11 to 18 years to complete themselves [59]. Both instruments were translated into Dutch and validated in The Netherlands [58,63]. Items for both instruments were generated from previously validated outcome instruments and expert opinion but not from patient interviews. The version for children aged 0 to 5 years was validated in a sample of 184 parents, and the version for children aged 5 to 18 years was validated in a sample of 186 parents and 86 adolescents (see Table 2).

Craniofacial

The following six instruments have been developed or adapted for use in children with various craniofacial conditions: (1) Quality of Life Instrument–Craniofacial Surgery (YQOL-CS) [84], (2) Youth Quality of Life Instrument–Facial Differences (YQOL-FD) [74,84], (3) Child Oral Health Quality of Life Questionnaire (COHQOL) [85,86,95,98], (4) Child Oral Health Impact Profile (COHIP) [99], (5) Pediatric Voice Outcome Survey (PVOS) [93], and (6) Pediatric Voice-Related Quality-of-Life (PVRQOL) survey [92].

Table 2: Condition-specific measures of QOL used with children who have conditions treated by plastic surgeons: content and psychometric information

Name of scale	Authors/year	Domains	Reliability	Validity	Responsiveness	References
Burns						
Burn Association/Shriners Hospitals for Children Burn Outcomes Questionnaire (BOQ), 0–5 years	Kazis et al, 2002	Play, language, fine motor skills, gross motor skills, behavior, family, pain/itching, appearance, satisfaction with care, concern/worry	Internal reliability (0.74–0.94), test-retest reliability (all but 3 domains >0.70)	Clinical validity: correlation of scores with clinical characteristics (eg, time since burn) Criterion validity: correlation of domain scores with child development measure	Over 6 months, 7 of 10 scales significantly different from no change	[87]
Burn Association/Shriners Hospitals for Children Burn Outcomes Questionnaire (BOQ), 5–18 years, parent form	Daltroy et al, 2000	Upper extremity function, physical function and sports, transfers and mobility, pain, itch, appearance, compliance, satisfaction with current state, emotional health, family disruption, parental concern, school re-entry	Internal reliability (0.82–0.93), test-retest reliability (0.67–0.99)	Within-scale analysis (correlations between domains were higher for similar constructs), correlations of domain scores with scores for generic QOL measure and with clinical variables	Not assessed	[59]
Burn Association/Shriners Hospitals for Children Burn Outcomes Questionnaire (BOQ), 11–18 years, adolescent form	Daltroy et al, 2000	Same domains as parent measure	Internal reliability (0.75–0.92), test-retest reliability not available	Within-scale analysis (correlations between domains were higher for similar constructs), correlations of domain scores with scores for generic QOL measure and with clinical variables	Not assessed	[59]

Instrument	Author	Content	Reliability	Validity	Responsiveness	Ref
Dutch Health Outcomes Burn Questionnaire (HOBQ), 0–4 years, parent form	van Baar et al, 2006	Same as American version	Internal reliability (0.69 [satisfaction]–0.96), test-retest reliability (all scales 0.7 or greater)	Correlation of domain scores with similar domains of a generic QOL measure and with clinical characteristics, ability to discriminate between children with burns of different severity	Not assessed	[63]
Dutch Burn Outcomes Questionnaire (BOQ), 5–18 years, parent form	van Baar et al, 2006	Same as American version	Internal reliability (0.69 [pain]–0.96), test-retest reliability (0.32 [satisfaction], rest 0.67–0.96)	Correlation with generic QOL measures, ability to discriminate between burns of different severity levels	Not assessed	[58]
Dutch Burn Outcomes Questionnaire (BOQ), 10–18 years, adolescent form	van Baar et al, 2006	Same as American version	Internal reliability (0.57 [emotional health]–0.96), test-retest reliability (0.32 [satisfaction], rest 0.67–0.96)	Correlation with generic QOL measures, ability to discriminate between burns of different severity levels	Not assessed	[58]
Craniofacial Youth Quality of Life Instrument-Craniofacial Surgery Module (YQOL-CS)	Edwards et al, 2005	Surgery	Not assessed	Not assessed	Not assessed	[84]
Youth Quality of Life Instrument-Facial Differences Module (YQOL-FD)	Patrick et al, 2007	Negative consequences, negative self-image, stigma, positive consequences, coping	Internal reliability (0.71–0.90), test-retest reliability (0.80–0.91)	Hypothesis testing: youth with more severe CFDs would have lower QOL, correlations between YQOL-FD and generic QOL measure, correlations between similar subscales of the YQOL-FD	Not assessed	[74]

(continued on next page)

Table 2: *(continued)*

Name of scale	Authors/year	Domains	Reliability	Validity	Responsiveness	References
Child Oral Health Quality of Life Questionnaire (COHQOL), Parent-Child Perceptions Questionnaire, 6–14 years	Jokovic et al, 2003	Oral symptoms, functional limitations, emotional well-being, social well-being	Internal reliability (0.69 [oral symptoms]–0.92. overall = 0.94), test-retest reliability (0.69 [oral symptoms]–0.85, overall = 0.85)	Hypothesis testing: poorer QOL scores would be for orofacial group, correlations of scores with clinical characteristics	Not assessed	[95]
Child Oral Health Quality of Life Questionnaire (COHQOL), Child Perceptions Questionnaire, 8–10 years	Jokovic et al, 2004	Oral symptoms, functional limitations, emotional well-being, social well-being	Internal reliability (0.63 [oral symptoms]–0.78, overall = 0.89), test-retest reliability (social well-being = 0.16, other scales 0.69 [emotional]–0.89, overall = 0.75)	Hypothesis testing: correlations between clinical characteristics and scores and lower QOL in orofacial group showed good construct validity but did not show discriminative validity	Not assessed	[86]
Child Oral Health Quality of Life Questionnaire (COHQOL), Child Perceptions Questionnaire, 11–14 years	Jokovic et al, 2002	Oral symptoms, functional limitations, emotional well-being, social well-being	Internal reliability (0.64 [oral symptoms]–0.86, overall = 0.91), test-retest reliability (0.79–0.88, overall = 0.90)	Ability to discriminate between groups, correlations between QOL scores and clinical characteristics and with global well-being ratings	Not assessed	[85]
Child Oral Health Quality of Life Questionnaire (COHQOL), Child Perceptions Questionnaire Short Forms, 11–14 years	Jokovic et al, 2006	Oral symptoms, functional limitations, emotional well-being, social well-being	Internal reliability (versions ranged from 0.71–0.83), test-retest reliability (versions ranged from 0.71–0.77)	Correlations between short- and long-form scores (0.87–0.98); hypothesis testing, lowest QOL in orofacial group; correlations of scores with clinical characteristics	Not assessed	[98]

Child Oral Health Impact Profile (COHIP)	Broder et al, 2007	Oral health, functional well-being, social/emotional well-being, school environment, self-image	Internal reliability (0.65 [school environment]–0.89, overall = 0.91), test-retest reliability (>0.58, overall = 0.84)	Discriminant and convergent validity supported by comparisons among and within the 4 groups of children	Not assessed	[99,100]
Pediatric Voice Outcomes Survey (PVOS)	Hartnick et al, 2002	Speaking voice, ability to be understood in a noisy area, interference with participation in social activities/school, strain during speech	Internal consistency reliability (0.57 [strain], 0.67 [speaking voice], 0.68 [participation], 0.74 [understanding in noisy area], overall = 0.86), test-retest reliability (weighted κ = 0.89)	Hypothesis testing: ability to discriminate between children before and after adenoidectomy	Not assessed	[93]
Pediatric Voice-Related Quality-of-Life (PVRQOL)	Boseley et al, 2006	Socioemotional, physical-functional	Internal consistency reliability (overall = 0.96), test-retest reliability (weighted κ = 0.80)	Correlations between PVRQOL and PVOS, ability to discriminate between children before and after adenoidectomy	Not assessed	[92]
Pectus excavatum Pectus Excavatum Evaluation Questionnaire (PEEQ), parent form, 8–18 years	Lawson et al, 2003	Psychosocial concerns, physical concerns, self-consciousness, caregiver concerns	Internal consistency (domains ranged from 0.7–0.8), test-retest reliability (9 of 13 items >0.70)	Not assessed	From before to at least 6 months after surgery, significant change occurred in all but 1 psychosocial item	[88]
Pectus Excavatum Evaluation Questionnaire (PEEQ), child form, 8–18 years	Lawson et al, 2003	Psychosocial concerns, physical concerns	Internal consistency (psychosocial = 0.8, physical = 0.9), test-retest reliability (9 of 12 items >0.70)	Not assessed	From before to at least 6 months after surgery, significant change occurred in all but 1 psychosocial item	[88]

The YQOL-CS and YQOL-FD modules are self-report instruments developed to measure QOL issues in adolescents aged 11 to 18 years with a broad range of craniofacial conditions [74,84]. Developed in two phases, the first phase described item generation and item reduction for both instruments. The second phase involved psychometric evaluation, but has only been reported for the YQOL-FD. Item generation for both measures involved a grounded theory approach with in-depth interviews conducted with 33 adolescents with a range of congenital and acquired craniofacial differences (CFDs) (burns, other trauma, birth marks, branchial arch disorders, isolated or syndromic craniosynostoses, cleft lip, cleft palate, or cleft lip and cleft palate). Additional items were developed from interviews and focus groups with parents of adolescents and young adults with CFDs, young adults with CFDs, and an expert panel. The authors also looked for existing relevant QOL instruments in the literature, but none existed. The original pool of 845 items was reduced to 125 items using investigator judgment, and these were presented to youth with CFDs, a panel, and parents for further item reduction. The YQOL-FD measure was field tested in a sample of 307 youth recruited from centers in the United States and United Kingdom [74]. A Spanish version of the questionnaire was completed by 48 youth. Formal item reduction testing led to refinement and reduction of the number of items to 30 perceptual and 18 contextual items across five domains.

The COHQOL was developed to assess QOL in children with a wide range of dental, oral, and orofacial disorders. The COHQOL includes the following versions: a parent version (P-CPQ) for children aged 6 to 14 years [95] and child versions for children aged 8 to 10 years (CPQ_{8-10}) [86] and 11 to 14 years (CPQ_{11-14}) [85]. In addition, 2 short-forms (8 and 16 items in length) have been developed for the CPQ_{11-14} [98]. The conceptual framework for the COHQOL was developed through a review of generic and disease-specific child QOL instruments. Item generation for the P-CPQ involved two phases. In the first, a preliminary pool of items was developed by abstracting items from existing questionnaires. In the second, face and content validity of the items was assessed and revised by a sample of clinicians and parents. A total of 47 items were then included in an item impact study with 208 parents, who were used to identify the items that they considered to be the most important. The final 31-item version of the questionnaire was administered to 231 parents to determine reliability and validity.

Items for the CPQ_{11-14} were also generated from existing oral health and child health status instruments. Comprehensiveness, relevance, and clarity were determined by an expert panel and a sample of parents. A revised item pool was refined through in-depth interviews with children. As with the P-CPQ, items for the final questionnaire were selected through an item impact study and performance of the final measure was determined in a psychometric study.

The CPQ_{8-10} was developed by adapting items from the CPQ_{11-14} and supplementing these with items developed on the basis of child development literature, experts, and parents. A convenience sample of children was used to assess readability, comprehension, and ease of administration.

The COHIP was developed to assess QOL in children aged 8 to 15 years with a range of dental, oral, and craniofacial disorders. Parallel forms are available for the child and parent/caregiver. This measure was designed to include positive (eg, confidence, attractiveness) as well as negative aspects of oral health-related QOL. The development of the COHIP involved six steps: (1) development of the initial pool of items; (2) initial face validity; (3) initial item impact; (4) revision of items, face validity of the revised instrument; (5) item impact of the revised instrument; and (6) factor analysis to identify conceptual domains. It is important to note that the initial item pool was composed of the 54 items developed by Jokovic and colleagues for the COHQOL described above. Through the various steps, some of these items were dropped and new ones added. The final questionnaire consisted of 34 items and five conceptually distinct subscales: oral health, functional well-being, social/emotional well-being, school environment, and self-image.

Two parent-proxy instruments were used to measure voice-related QOL in children with otolaryngologic diagnoses. Both instruments were adapted from adult instruments, and therefore did not involve children in item generation or reduction. In the first, Hartnick [102] modified the Voice Outcome Survey (VOS) to create a measure called the Pediatric Voice Outcome Survey (PVOS). This four-item measure was validated in a sample of children with and without tracheotomies. To broaden the applicability of the PVOS to children with other vocal disorders, the instrument was included by Hartnick and colleagues [93] in a study of 385 parents of children aged 2 to 18 years with a range of conditions, including velopharyngeal insufficiency, subglottic stenosis, vocal cord nodules, reflux laryngitis, vocal cord paralysis, obstructive sleep apnea, adenotonsillar hypertrophy, otitis media, and sinus disorder.

Boseley and colleagues [92] validated the 10-item PVRQOL survey in a study of 104 parents of children aged 2 to 18 years with a variety of otolaryngologic diagnoses, including velopharyngeal insufficiency, dysphonia, adenotonsillar hypertrophy, otitis media, and sinus disorder.

Pectus excavatum

The Pectus Excavatum Evaluation Questionnaire (PEEQ) was developed to measure QOL issues in children before and after surgical repair of pectus excavatum [88]. The instrument can be administered before and after surgery, and there is a 12-item child version for children aged 8 to 18 years and a 13-item parent version. Item generation involved expert input but not literature review or patient interviews. This study used a small sample of parents (n = 24) and children (n = 19) to evaluate the instrument's psychometric properties.

Discussion

In this section on outcome measures, the authors have identified several methodologic and conceptual issues specific to measuring outcomes in pediatric patients undergoing plastic surgery. In identifying already developed condition-specific measures of QOL, the authors' review highlights where future research in instrument development is needed. The authors found eight pediatric condition-specific measures developed to assess outcome in children with burns, craniofacial conditions, and pectus excavatum. Six of these measures (exceptions were the PVOS and PVRQOL) included a child self-report measure. Given that children often report a QOL that is different from that reported by their parents, the development of self-report measures is highly important. Although all eight instruments underwent some degree of formal development and validation, only one (the YQOL-FD) followed the gold standard guidelines for health outcomes instrument development summarized by Cano and colleagues [81] and can be highly recommended. This instrument was lacking only in terms of information about its ability to detect change over time.

For seven instruments, formal tests for item reduction (eg, item redundancy, tests of scaling assumptions) and psychometric analysis (eg, item total correlations, responsiveness) were often not assessed by the developers. Of particular concern is that only the YQOL-FD and the YQOL-CS involved children in the item generation process. In-depth qualitative interviews are an important component of item generation because they produce questions that are relevant and important to patients. Expert opinion or literature review alone cannot be expected to uncover all the issues that patients consider important. Without adequate input from patients, those questions that matter most to them may remain unasked.

Another concern is that two questionnaires (ie, PVOS and PVRQOL) represent adaptations from adult instruments. In adapting an adult measure for use with children, an important question is whether the domains used to assess QOL in adults are appropriate to assess QOL in children [43]. Adult measures may fail to tap the specific aspects of QOL that are important to children, and the extent to which this is the case is unclear for the PVOS and PVRQOL.

It is important that QOL measures be developed and validated for specific target populations. Several instruments identified in this review were designed to measure QOL concerns of a heterogeneous sample of children, such as the YQOL-FD, which is applicable to children with a wide range of craniofacial conditions. It is possible that these broader plastic surgery measures of QOL may not be sensitive enough to the concerns of a particular subgroup of patients (eg, patients who have cleft lip and palate) and that the development of a more specific measure may be called for.

For a researcher wanting to measure QOL in a pediatric plastic surgery study, it is crucial to inspect carefully the QOL domains of any candidate generic or condition-specific measure to ensure that the content of the instrument is appropriate for the research about to be undertaken. The authors found that the YQOL-FD, COHQOL, and COHIP can be used to measure QOL in children with cleft lip and palate, but an inspection of the content of each measure shows that each is based on different conceptual models of QOL. Similarly, although the PVOS and PVRQOL can be used to measure QOL in children with velopharyngeal insufficiency, the instruments differ in content and length.

Summary

Pediatric patients who undergo plastic surgery represent a broad heterogeneous group of patients. There are a variety of study designs that have been used to date to measure outcome in pediatric patients undergoing plastic surgery. Traditional outcome measures (eg, complication rates, other quantifiable clinical data) are not sufficient on their own to assess outcome in this specialty. Given that surgery can have a major impact on the QOL of children and their families, it is important that research include broader measures of outcome. Although QOL instruments provide a means to assess child health more comprehensively than has previously been the case, the authors' review of the literature shows that clinically meaningful and psychometrically sound plastic surgery–specific measures of QOL are lacking. Only one condition-specific QOL measure can be recommended without hesitation (ie, YQOL-FD). Although it may not be feasible or practical because of the small size of some surgical subgroups to develop condition-specific measures for all the different problems treated by pediatric plastic surgeons, there is certainly room for the development of more psychometrically sound measures of QOL for the main pediatric plastic surgery conditions. The authors would suggest that a coordinated research effort is needed to identify the most common plastic surgical procedures performed in children and to use sound methodology to develop measures for these conditions that are meaningful and responsive to surgical change. Such an approach should help to ensure that psychometrically sound measures of the impact of surgery from the child's perspective are available to future research endeavors.

Acknowledgments

Anne Klassen is a recipient of Canadian Institute of Health Research career award. The authors acknowledge the contribution of Maureen Rice and Emma Love for their help with the systematic review.

References

[1] Millard DR. Refinements in rotation-advancement cleft lip technique. Plast Reconstr Surg 1964;33(1):26–38.
[2] Mulliken JB. Principles and techniques of bilateral complete cleft lip repair. Plast Reconstr Surg 1985;75(4):477–87.
[3] Furlow LT. Cleft palate repair by double opposing Z-plasty. Plast Reconstr Surg 1986;78(6):724–38.
[4] Tessier P. The definitive plastic surgical treatment of the severe facial deformities of craniofacial dysostosis. Crouzon's and Apert's diseases. Plast Reconstr Surg 1971;48(5):419–42.
[5] Bradley JP, Gabbay JS, Taub PJ, et al. Monobloc advancement by distraction osteogenesis decreases morbidity and relapse. Plast Reconstr Surg 2006;118(7):1585–97.
[6] Tanzer RC. Total reconstruction of the external ear. Plast Reconstr Surg 1959;23(1):1–15.
[7] Brent B. The correction of microtia with autogenous cartilage grafts: I. The classic deformity. Plast Reconstr Surg 1980;66(1):1–12.
[8] Nagata S. A new method of total reconstruction of the auricle for microtia. Plast Reconstr Surg 1993;92(2):187–201.
[9] Alderman BW, Bradley CM, Greene C, et al. Increased risk of craniosynostosis with maternal cigarette smoking during pregnancy. Teratology 1994;50(1):13–8.
[10] Speltz ML, Kapp-Simon K, Collett B, et al. Neurodevelopment of infants with single-suture craniosynostosis: presurgery comparisons with case-matched controls. Plast Reconstr Surg 2007;119(6):1874–81.
[11] Romitti PA, Sun L, Honein MA, et al. The national birth defects prevention study. Maternal periconceptional alcohol consumption and risk of orofacial clefts. Am J Epidemiol 2007;166(7):775–85.
[12] Carmichael SL, Shaw GM, Yang W, et al. Maternal stressful life events and risks of birth defects. Epidemiology 2007;18(3):356–61.
[13] Wilcox AJ, Lie RT, Solvoll K, et al. Folic acid supplements and risk of facial clefts: national population based case-control study. BMJ 2007;334(7591):464–70.
[14] Chung KC, Kowalski CP, Kim HM, et al. Maternal cigarette smoking during pregnancy and the risk of having a child with cleft lip/palate. Plast Reconstr Surg 2000;105(2):485–9.
[15] Man LX, Chang B. Maternal cigarette smoking during pregnancy increases the risk of having a child with a congenital digital anomaly. Plast Reconstr Surg 2006;117(1):301–8.
[16] McComb HK, Coghlan BA. Primary repair of the unilateral cleft lip nose: completion of a longitudinal study. Cleft Palate Craniofac J 1996;33(1):23–30.
[17] Berkowitz S, Mejia M, Bystrik A. A comparison of the effects of the Latham-Millard procedure with those of a conservative treatment approach for dental occlusion and facial aesthetics in unilateral and bilateral complete cleft lip and palate: part I. Dental occlusion. Plast Reconstr Surg 2004;113(1):1–18.
[18] Shetye PR, Grayson BH, Mackool RJ, et al. Long-term stability and growth following unilateral mandibular distraction in growing children with craniofacial microsomia. Plast Reconstr Surg 2006;118(4):985–95.
[19] Brent B. Auricular repair with autogenous rib cartilage grafts: two decades of experience with 600 cases. Plast Reconstr Surg 1992;90(3):355–74 [discussion 375–6].
[20] McCarthy JG, Glasberg SB, Cutting CB, et al. Twenty-year experience with early surgery for craniosynostosis: I. Isolated craniofacial synostosis-results and unsolved problems. Plast Reconstr Surg 1995;96(2):272–83.
[21] Becker DB, Petersen JD, Kane AA, et al. Speech, cognitive, and behavioral outcomes in nonsyndromic craniosynostosis. Plast Reconstr Surg 2005;116(2):400–7.
[22] Prahl C, Kuijpers-Jagtman AM, van't Hof MA, et al. A randomised prospective clinical trial into the effect of infant orthopaedics on maxillary arch dimensions in unilateral cleft lip and palate (Dutchcleft). Eur J Oral Sci 2001;109(5):297–305.

[23] Prahl C, Kuijpers-Jagtman AM, van't Hof MA, et al. A randomised prospective clinical trial of the effect of infant orthopaedics in unilateral cleft lip and palate: prevention of collapse of the alveolar segments (Dutchcleft). Cleft Palate Craniofac J 2003;40(4):337–42.

[24] Prahl C, Kuijpers-Jagtman AM, van't Hof MA, et al. The effects of infant orthopedics on the occlusion of the deciduous dentition in children with complete unilateral cleft lip and palate (Dutchcleft). Cleft Palate Craniofac J 2004; 41(6):633–41.

[25] Prahl C, Kuijpers-Jagtman AM, van't Hof MA, et al. Infant orthopedics in UCLP: effect on feeding, weight, and length: a randomized clinical trial (Dutchcleft). Cleft Palate Craniofac J 2005;42(2):171–7.

[26] Abyholm F, D'Antonio L, Davidson Ward SL, et al. Pharyngeal flap and sphincteroplasty for velopharyngeal insufficiency have equal outcome at 1 year postoperatively: results of a randomized trial. Cleft Palate Craniofac J 2005; 42(5):501–11.

[27] Senders CW, Di Mauro SM, Brodie HA, et al. The efficacy of perioperative steroid therapy in pediatric primary palatoplasty. Cleft Palate Craniofac J 1999;36(4):340–4.

[28] Fearon JA, Weinthal J. The use of recombinant erythropoietin in the reduction of blood transfusion rates in craniosynostosis repair in infants and children. Plast Reconstr Surg 2002;109(7): 2190–6.

[29] Glenny AM, Hooper L, Shaw WC, et al. Feeding interventions for growth and development in infants with cleft lip, cleft palate or cleft lip and palate. Cochrane Database of Systematic Reviews 2004;3: CD003315.

[30] Liao YF, Mars M. Hard palate repair timing and facial growth in cleft lip and palate: a systematic review. Cleft Palate Craniofac J 2006;43(5): 563–70.

[31] Bialocerkowski AE, Vladusic SL, Howell SM. Conservative interventions for positional plagiocephaly: a systematic review. Dev Med Child Neurol 2005;47(8):563–70.

[32] Meling TR, Hans-Erik H, Per S, et al. Le Fort III distraction osteogenesis in syndromal craniosynostosis. J Craniofac Surg 2006;17(1): 28–39.

[33] Hollier LH Jr, Higuera S, Stal S, et al. Distraction rate and latency: factors in the outcome of pediatric mandibular distraction. Plast Reconstr Surg 2006;117(7):2333–6.

[34] Iannetti G, Fadda T, Agrillo A, et al. LeFort III advancement with and without osteogenesis distraction. J Craniofac Surg 2006;17(3):536–43.

[35] Wu JK, Bisdorff A, Gelbert F, et al. Auricular arteriovenous malformation: evaluation, management, and outcome. Plast Reconstr Surg 2005; 115(4):985–95.

[36] Greene AK, Burrows PE, Smith L, et al. Periorbital lymphatic malformation: clinical course and management in 42 patients. Plast Reconstr Surg 2005;115(1):22–30.

[37] Yamada T, Mori Y, Minami K, et al. Three-dimensional analysis of facial morphology in normal Japanese children as control data for cleft surgery. Cleft Palate Craniofac J 2002; 39(5):517–26.

[38] Phillips JG. Photo-cephalometric analysis in treatment planning for surgical correction of facial disharmonies. J Maxillofac Surg 1978;6(3): 174–9.

[39] Guyatt GH, Veldhuyzen Van Zanten SJO, Feeny DH, et al. Measuring quality of life in clinical trials: a taxonomy and review. CMAJ 1989;140(12):1441–8.

[40] Spieth LE, Harris CV. Assessment of health related quality of life in children and adolescents: an integrative review. J Pediatr Psychol 1996; 21(2):175–93.

[41] Connolly MA, Johnson JA. Measuring quality of life in paediatric patients. Pharmacoeconomics 1999;16(6):605–25.

[42] Eiser C, Mohay H, Morse R. The measurement of quality of life in young children. Child Care Health Dev 2000;26(5):401–14.

[43] Eiser C, Morse R. Quality-of-life measures in chronic diseases of childhood. Health Technol Assess 2001;5(4):1–157.

[44] Harding L. Children's quality of life assessments: a review of generic and health related quality of life measures completed by children and adolescents. Clin Psychol Psychother 2001;8(2):79–96.

[45] Schmidt LJ, Garrat AM, Fitzpatrick R. Child/parent-assessed population health outcome measures: a structured review. Child Care Health Dev 2002;28(3):227–37.

[46] Clarke S, Eiser C. The measurement of health-related quality of life (QOL) in paediatric clinical trials: a systematic review. Health Qual Life Outcomes 2004;2:66.

[47] Matza LS, Swensen AR, Flood EM, et al. Assessment of health-related quality of life in children: a review of conceptual, methodological, and regulatory issues. Value Health 2004;7(1):79–92.

[48] Rajmil L, Herdman M, Fernandez De Sanmamed M, et al. Generic health-related quality of life instruments in children and adolescents: a qualitative analysis of content. J Adolesc Health 2004;34(1):37–45.

[49] De Civita M, Regier D, Alamgir AH, et al. Evaluating health-related-quality-of-life studies in paediatric populations. Some conceptual, methodological and developmental considerations and recent applications. Pharmacoeconomics 2006;23(7):659–85.

[50] Cremeens J, Eiser E, Blades M. Characteristics of health-related self-report measures for children aged three to eight years: a review of the literature. Qual Life Res 2006;15(4):739–54.

[51] Davis E, Waters E, Mackinnon A, et al. Paediatric quality of life instruments: a review of the

[52] Ravens-Sieberer U, Erhart M, Wille N, et al. Generic health-related quality-of-life assessment in children and adolescents. Pharmacoeconomics 2006;24(12):1199–220.
[53] Raat H, Mohangoo AD, Grootenhuis MA. Pediatric health-related quality of life questionnaires in clinical trials. Curr Opin Allergy Clin Immunol 2006;6(3):180–5.
[54] Starfield B, Riley A, Green B, et al. The child health and illness profile. A population-based measure of health. Med Care 1995;33(5): 553–66.
[55] Slifer KJ, Beck M, Amari A, et al. Self-concept and satisfaction with physical appearance in youth with and without oral clefts. Child Health Care 2003;32(2):81–101.
[56] Landgraf JM, Abetz L, Ware JE. The CHQ user's manual. Second printing. Boston: HealthAct; 1999.
[57] Warschausky S, Kay JB, Buchman S, et al. Health-related quality of life in children with craniofacial anomalies. Plast Reconstr Surg 2002;110(2):409–14.
[58] van Baar ME, Essink-Bot ML, Oen IM, et al. Reliability and validity of the Dutch version of the American Burn Association/Shriners Hospital for Children Burn Outcomes Questionnaire (5–18 years of age). J Burn Care Res 2006; 27(6):790–802.
[59] Daltroy LH, Liang MH, Phillips CB, et al. American Burn Association/Shriners Hospitals for Children Burn Outcomes Questionnaire: construction and psychometric properties. [erratum appears in J Burn Care Rehabil 2000 Mar-Apr;21(2):170]. J Burn Care Rehabil 2000; 21(1:Pt 1):29–39.
[60] Lam MCW, Klassen AF, Montgomery CJ, et al. Quality of life outcomes following surgical correction of pectus excavatuum: a comparison of the Ravitch and Nuss procedure. J Pediatr Surg, in press.
[61] Klassen AF, Landgraf JM, Lee SK. Health related quality of life in 3 and 4 year old children: preliminary findings about a new questionnaire. Health Qual Life Outcomes 2003;1(1): 81.
[62] Raat H, Landgraf JM, Oostenbrink R, et al. Reliability and validity of the Infant and Toddler Quality of Life Questionnaire (ITQOL) in a general population and respiratory disease sample. Qual Life Res 2007;16(3):445–60.
[63] van Baar ME, Essink-Bot ML, Oen IM, et al. Reliability and validity of the health outcomes burn questionnaire for infants and children in The Netherlands. Burns 2006;32(3):357–65.
[64] Ravens-Sieberer U, Bullinger M. Assessing health-related quality of life in chronically ill children with the German KINDL: first psychometric and content analytical results. Qual Life Res 1998;7(5):399–407.
[65] Bressmann T, Sader R, Ravens-Sieberer U, et al. Quality of life research in patients with cleft lip and palate: preliminary results. Mund Kiefer Gesichtschir 1999;3(3):134–9.
[66] Varni JW, Burwinkle TM, Seid M, et al. The PedsQL 4.0 as a pediatric population health measure: feasibility, reliability, and validity. Ambul Rediatr 2003;3:329–41.
[67] Damiano PC, Tyle MC, Romitti PA, et al. Health-related quality of life among preadolescent children with oral clefts: the mother's perspective. Pediatrics 2007;120(2):e283–90.
[68] Vogels T, Verrips GH, Koopman HM, et al. TACQOL Manual: Parent and Child Form, Leiden, Netherlands: Leiden Center for Child Health and Paediatrics LUMC-TNO; 2000.
[69] Graf A, Landolt MA, Mori AC, et al. Quality of life and psychological adjustment in children and adolescents with neurofibromatosis type 1. J Pediatr 2006;149(3):348–53.
[70] Boltshauser E, Ludwig S, Dietrich F, et al. Sagittal craniosynostosis: cognitive development, behaviour, and quality of life in unoperated children. Neuropediatrics 2003;34(6):293–300.
[71] Landolt MA, Grubenmann S, Meuli M. Family impact greatest: predictors of quality of life and psychological adjustment in pediatric burn survivors. J Trauma 2002;53(6):1146–51.
[72] Topolski TD, Edwards TC, Patrick DL. User's manual and interpretation guide for the youth quality of life (YQOL) instruments. Seattle (WA): University of Washington; 2002.
[73] Topolski TD, Edwards TC, Patrick DL. Quality of life: how do adolescents with facial differences compare with other adolescents? Cleft Palate Craniofac J 2005;42(1):25–32.
[74] Patrick DL, Topolski TD, Edwards TC, et al. Measuring the quality of life of youth with facial differences. Cleft Palate Craniofac J 2007; 44(5):538–47.
[75] Fayers PM, Machin D. Quality of life: assessment, analysis, and interpretation. New York: John Wiley; 2000.
[76] Food and Drug Administration. Patient reported outcome measures: use in medical product development to support labeling claims. Available at: http://www.fda.gov/cber/gdlns/prolbl.pdf. Accessed July 19, 2007.
[77] Davis E, Nicolas C, Waters E, et al. Parent-proxy and child self-reported health-related quality of life: using qualitative methods to explain the discordance. Qual Life Res 2007;16(5):863–71.
[78] Ungar WJ, Mirabelli C, Cousins M, et al. A qualitative analysis of a dyad approach to health-related quality of life measurement in children with asthma. Soc Sci Med 2006;63(9):2354–66.
[79] Riley AW. Evidence that school-age children can self-report on their health. Ambul Pediatr 2004; 4(4):371–6.

[80] McGrath PA, Seifert CE, Speechley KN, et al. A new analogue scale for assessing children's pain: an initial validation study. Pain 1996; 64(3):435–43.

[81] Cano SJ, Browne JP, Lamping DL, et al. The Patient Outcomes of Surgery-Hand/Arm (POS-Hand/Arm): a new patient-based outcome measure. J Hand Surg [Br] 2004;29(5):477–85.

[82] Scientific Advisory Committee of the Medical Outcomes Trust. Assessing health status and quality of life instruments: attributes and review criteria. Qual Life Res 2002;11(3): 193–205.

[83] Boseley ME, Hartnick CJ. Assessing the outcome of surgery to correct velopharyngeal insufficiency with the pediatric voice outcomes survey. Int J Pediatr Otorhinolaryngol 2004; 68(11):1429–33.

[84] Edwards TC, Patrick DL, Topolski TD, et al. Approaches to craniofacial-specific quality of life assessment in adolescents. Cleft Palate Craniofac J 2005;42(1):19–24.

[85] Jokovic A, Locker D, Stephens M, et al. Validity and reliability of a questionnaire for measuring child oral-health-related quality of life. J Dent Res 2002;81(7):459–63.

[86] Jokovic A, Locker D, Tompson B, et al. Questionnaire for measuring oral health-related quality of life in eight- to ten-year-old children. Pediatr Dent 2004;26(6):512–8.

[87] Kazis LE, Liang MH, Lee A, et al. The development, validation, and testing of a health outcomes burn questionnaire for infants and children 5 years of age and younger: American Burn Association/Shriners Hospitals for Children. J Burn Care Rehabil 2002;23(3): 196–207.

[88] Lawson ML, Cash TF, Akers R, et al. A pilot study of the impact of surgical repair on disease-specific quality of life among patients with pectus excavatum. J Pediatr Surg 2003; 38(6):916–8.

[89] Locker D, Jokovic A, Tompson B. Health-related quality of life of children aged 11 to 14 years with orofacial conditions. Cleft Palate Craniofac J 2005;42(3):260–6.

[90] Weber TR. Further experience with the operative management of asphyxiating thoracic dystrophy after pectus repair. J Pediatr Surg 2005; 40(1):170–3.

[91] Strauss RP, Ramsey BL, Edwards TC, et al. Stigma experiences in youth with facial differences: a multi-site study of adolescents and their mothers. Orthod Craniofac Res 2007;10(2): 96–103.

[92] Boseley ME, Cunningham M, Volk MS, et al. Validation of the Pediatric Voice-Related Quality-of-Life survey. Arch Otolaryngol Head Neck Surg 2006;132(7):717–20.

[93] Hartnick CJ, Volk MS, Cunningham M. Establishing normative voice-related quality of life scores within the pediatric otolaryngology population. Arch Otolaryngol Head Neck Surg 2003;129(10):1090–3.

[94] Jokovic A, Locker D, Stephens M, et al. Agreement between mothers and children aged 11–14 years in rating child oral health-related quality of life. Community Dent Oral Epidemiol 2003;31(5):335–43.

[95] Jokovic A, Locker D, Stephens M, et al. Measuring parental perceptions of child oral health-related quality of life. J Public Health Dent 2003; 63(2):67–72.

[96] Jokovic A, Locker D, Guyatt G. How well do parents know their children? Implications for proxy reporting of child health-related quality of life. Qual Life Res 2004;13(7): 1297–307.

[97] Jokovic A, Locker D, Guyatt G. What do children's global ratings of oral health and well-being measure? Community Dent Oral Epidemiol 2005;33(3):205–11.

[98] Jokovic A, Locker D, Guyatt G. Short forms of the Child Perceptions Questionnaire for 11–14-year-old children (CPQ11-14): development and initial evaluation. Health Qual Life Outcomes 2006;4(4):1–9.

[99] Broder HL, McGrath C, Cisnero GJ. Questionnaire development: face validity and item impact testing of the Child Oral Health Impact Profile. Community Dent Oral Epidemiol 2007; 35(Suppl 1):8–19.

[100] Broder HL, Wilson-Genderson M. Reliability and convergent and discriminant validity of the Child Oral Health Impact Profile (COHIP Child's version). Community Dent Oral Epidemiol 2007;35(Suppl 1):20–31.

[101] Wilson-Genderson M, Broder HL, Phillips C. Concordance between caregiver and child reports of children's oral health-related quality of life. Community Dent Oral Epidemiol 2007;35(Suppl 1):32–40.

[102] Hartnick C. Validation of a pediatric voice quality of life instrument: the Pediatric Voice Outcome Survey (PVOS). Arch Otolaryngol Head Neck Surg 2002;128(8):919–22.

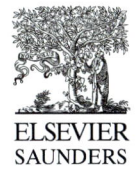

Clinical Research in Aesthetic Surgery

Shim Ching, MSc, MD, FRCSC, FACS[a], Gloria Rockwell, MD, MSc, FRCSC[b], Achilleas Thoma, MD, MSc, FRCS(C), FACS[c,d,e,*], Martin M. Antony, PhD, ABPP[f]

- Study design in aesthetic surgery
- Measurement of outcomes in aesthetic surgery
- Recent outcomes studies
- Summary
- References

The nature of aesthetic surgery, the creation of beauty, will always be a difficult subject for study. In no other field of surgery is artistry so apparent and results consequently so difficult to measure. Perhaps these are the reasons why advancements in aesthetic surgery clinical research have been difficult to achieve.

Research in aesthetic surgery cannot rely upon traditional measures of surgical success, such as mortality, morbidity, and physiologic function. Conventionally, visual evaluations of selected pre- and postoperative photographs form the basis of aesthetic surgery assessments. While photographs will always play an important role in aesthetic surgery, their use in conducting meaningful clinical research is limited because of the introduction of bias.

Our group in 2003 published a comprehensive review of the literature to determine the most appropriate methods to conduct clinical research in aesthetic surgery [1]. Appropriate patient assessment tools were identified. Our review concluded that outcomes-based methods show the most promise for future research in aesthetic surgery. Since that time, while some studies have used an outcomes-based approach, the potential of outcomes-based research in aesthetic surgery has not been reached.

Outcomes research seeks to study the effect of medical interventions by examining the preferences, experiences, and values of patients [2]. The patient's own assessment of outcomes in aesthetic surgery is especially pertinent because the patient's perception of outcome is often the key factor in determining the success of aesthetic interventions. Outcomes research recognizes that patient perspectives are essential in judging the results of treatment.

---

[a] Department of Surgery, University of Hawaii, 550 South Beretania Street, Suite 603, Honolulu, HI 96813, USA
[b] Department of Surgery, Division of Plastic Surgery, University of Ottawa, 1919 Riverside Drive, Suite 401, Ottawa, ON K1H 1A2, Canada
[c] Department of Surgery, Division of Plastic Surgery, McMaster University, St. Joseph's Healthcare, 50 Charlton Avenue East, Hamilton, ON L8N 486, Canada
[d] Department of Clinical Epidemiology and Biostatistics, McMaster University, 1200 Main Street West, Hamilton, ON L8N 3Z5, Canada
[e] Surgical Outcomes Research Centre (SOURCE), McMaster University, St. Joseph's Healthcare, 50 Charlton Avenue East, Hamilton, ON L8N 4A6, Canada
[f] Department of Psychology, Ryerson University, 350 Victoria Street, Toronto, ON MB5 2K3, Canada
* Corresponding author. 206 James Street South, Suite 101, Hamilton, ON L8P 3A9, Canada
E-mail address: athoma@mcmaster.ca (A. Thoma).

There are many benefits for adopting outcomes research methods in aesthetic surgery. Commonly adopted outcome measurement scales could form the basis for comparing surgical techniques. The effects of aesthetic surgery on patients could be ascertained and quantified. The benefit of these procedures could be compared with other medical interventions to demonstrate their positive effects on the quality of life (QOL) of patients.

Unfortunately, few studies have used outcome research methods in aesthetic surgery. Our review discusses the research designs and methods that have been used in aesthetic surgery and suggests future directions for clinical research.

Study design in aesthetic surgery

The typical study design appearing in the aesthetic surgery literature is a descriptive presentation of a case series of a single surgeon (usually an "expert"). Complications may be listed. Preoperative and postoperative photographs of selected cases are the main focus for measuring the success of the surgical intervention in question. Generally, only favorable results are presented.

While, the safety of a technique and the skill of the surgeon may be ascertained from this type of study, few other conclusions can be drawn. There may be a strong bias for surgeons to present only successful outcomes. The effect of a surgical intervention on an entire group of individuals cannot be examined. Because different surgical procedures are not compared, the effectiveness of new techniques is never known. As is apparent from these shortcomings, these case series represent the least favorable study design, forming essentially an opinion of a respected authority, based on clinical experience. This study design is at the bottom of the pyramid of the hierarchy of evidence. (See the article by Sprague, McKay, and Thoma in this issue.)

One approach to improving research study design has been to stratify the quality of a study on the basis of degree of freedom from various biases inherent in clinical research. The quality of the study in question is assigned a hierarchical rating termed the "level of evidence."

Given that aesthetic surgery examines patients subjected to surgical interventions, prospective cohort studies (where consecutive patients are followed over time) and randomized controlled trials (RCTs) are appropriate study designs. Eventually, meta-analyses or qualitative systematic reviews of these RCTs or cohort studies will likely represent the highest levels of evidence possible in aesthetic surgery. (See the articles by Thoma, Sprague, Temple, and Archibald; and Haines, McKnight, Duku, Perry, and Thoma in this issue.)

The assessment of surgical outcomes is a critical component of study design. The selection of appropriate tools to assess patient outcome is crucial.

Measurement of outcomes in aesthetic surgery

In outcomes research, patient questionnaires are used to determine the effect of interventions. Various interchangeable terms are used for these questionnaires, such as scales, instruments, and measures.

Key factors that should be considered in the evaluation of outcome instruments are validity, reliability, and responsiveness to change. These attributes ensure that the instrument is appropriate, accurate, and sensitive in examining the outcome in question. By demonstrating validity and reliability, outcome instruments show that they have undergone rigorous testing, forming the basis for widespread acceptance of an instrument.

The term validity encompasses many related concepts. Face validity refers to whether the scale's items seem, on the surface, to reflect the construct being measured. For example, a measure of patient satisfaction would be said to have adequate face validity if the items ask about patient satisfaction. Content validity refers to whether the content of a scale encompasses the relevant aspects of the construct purported to be measured. For example, a broad measure of QOL might be expected to include items measuring a wide range of life domains, including work, relationships, and health. Predictive validity refers to whether a measure can predict a patient's response on a measure of some related construct. For example, a measure of patient satisfaction with aesthetic surgery should predict the likelihood of a patient seeking repeated surgeries in the future to "correct" the original procedure. Convergent validity refers to whether scores on a particular measure correlate with scores on other measures that measure the same construct, whereas discriminate validity refers to the tendency of scores on a particular measure to be uncorrelated with scores on other measures that are believed to assess a theoretically unrelated construct.

Reliability refers to whether a scale yields the same results when subjected to repeated measurements under different conditions. Many aspects of reliability can be examined. Internal consistency refers to the correlation among items in the measure, and is usually expressed as Cronbach's alpha. Stability refers to the reproducibility of a measure. This can be assessed in a variety of ways. Interobserver reliability measures the degree of agreement between different observers, expressed as Cohen's kappa. Intraobserver reliability examines the agreement between observations made by the same evaluator on two different occasions (intraclass coefficient). Test–retest reliability examines the agreement between observations on the same patient on two occasions separated by a time interval (Spearman-Brown coefficient). Although opinions vary, accepted values for internal consistency usually exceed 0.7 but should be no greater than 0.9 to avoid redundancy, whereas stability measures should be greater than 0.5 [3].

Methods of critical and systematic evaluation have been proposed to adequately evaluate outcome instruments [4]. Evaluations of outcome instruments should consider:

- How feasible is the scale to administer? Is the time and effort required to administer the scale realistic for the patient and researcher?
- Does the scale demonstrate appropriate validity with respect to aesthetic surgery?
- Has the scale been shown to display acceptable reliability?
- Has the scale been tested on surgical subjects and, if so, what is the scale's ability to detect changes resulting from surgery?
- Can the quantitative score of an instrument be easily understood?

In our previous review [1], we identified psychometric instruments and QOL measures as the outcome tools showing the most promise in aesthetic surgery clinical research. These instruments and some newer tools are summarized in Table 1. The Multidimensional Body-States Relations Questionnaire (MBSRQ) is a psychometric assessment of multiple aspects of body image and has undergone rigorous evaluation. Health-related QOL (HRQL), a component of a person's overall QOL, comprises all areas specific to health. That is, physical, emotional, psychological, social, and cognitive well-being; ability to function in specific roles in life; general abilities; relationships; perceptions; life satisfaction; and overall well-being. HRQL is based on each patient's appraisal of his or her current level of functioning and satisfaction with it in comparison with what the patient perceives to be the ideal level of functioning [6,7].

QOL measurement tools can be classified as either health status or preference-based instruments. Health status instruments divide QOL into several domains and provide a score in each of the domains. The most widely used generic (ie, applicable to subjects with various diseases) health status QOL instrument is the Medical Outcomes Study Short Form-36 (SF-36) [8]. The Derriford Scale (DAS59) is a condition-specific QOL instrument developed specifically for aesthetic surgery [9]. The Breast Evaluation Questionnaire is a newly developed, validated, and reliable scale that may be appropriate for breast-augmentation patients [10]. An advantage of these condition-specific instruments is that they may be more sensitive to changes after surgery and they can provide detailed information regarding the condition in question.

Preference-based QOL instruments elicit patients' valuations for their current health state. The instruments generate a single QOL value expressed on a zero to one ratio scale, where zero represents the value of death and one represents the value of perfect health. This valuation of a health state is also known as a "utility," a concept developed by economists to indicate the strength of an individual's preference. Preference-based QOL measurements, increasingly common in the medical literature, have the advantage of allowing comparisons of health status across many different conditions [11]. Another advantage of preference-based instruments is their usefulness for conducting economic analyses to compare the cost of a surgical intervention with its effectiveness. (See the article by Thoma, Strumas, Rockwell, and McKnight in this issue.)

Examples of preference-based instruments include the EuroQol (EQ-5D) [12] and the Health Utilities Index (HUI) [13]. A disadvantage of preference-based instruments is that they may be unable to detect change in individuals because they were designed for population assessment. Guyatt and colleagues [14] have recommended including both a generic and a condition-specific instrument in outcomes studies to ensure the detection of changes following medical interventions.

Recent outcomes studies

Sarwer and colleagues [15] used the MBSRQ prospectively on a group of women undergoing cosmetic surgery. Mixed improvements in some aspects of body image were seen, but this may be due to the variety of different surgical procedures that the study group had experienced.

Bolton and colleagues [16] prospectively examined 30 abdominoplasty patients with the MBSRQ and found positive changes in instrument components related to body area satisfaction, body exposure, and sexual relations. Unfortunately, the study was limited to a 2-month follow-up.

Studies of women following breast reduction are notable for the use of outcomes instruments. Hermans and colleagues [17] studied 84 women after reduction mammoplasty, with a mean follow-up of 25 months. A control group of women waiting for reduction mammoplasty was used. The SF-36 showed a significant increase in QOL and the DAS-59 showed higher scores in various domains. The EQ-5D showed a significantly marked increase after surgery.

Table 1: Summary of selected outcome instruments

Name	Investigators	Numerical characteristics[a]	No. of items[b]	Applications of method	Method of administration (time)	Reliability: thoroughness[c]	Reliability: results[d]	Validity: thoroughness[c]	Validity: results[d]	Sensitivity to change[e]
Multidimensional Body-States Relations Questionnaire (MBSRQ)	Cash [5]	Interval	69	Psychometric, body image, general	Self-administered (10 min)	+++	+++	+++	+++	++
Derriford Appearance Scale (DAS 59)	Harris and Carr [9]	Interval	59	QOL, general	Self-administered (10 min)	+++	+++	+++	+++	+++
Breast Evaluation Questionnaire (BEQ)	Anderson et al [10]	Interval	55	QOL, breast-specific	Self-administered (10 min)	+++	+++	+++	+++	+++
Short Form 36 (SF-36)	Ware [8]	Interval	36	QOL, general	Self-administered (10 min)	+++	+++	+++	+++	+
EuroQol (EQ-5D)	EuroQol Group [12]	Interval	6	QOL, general	Self-administered (5 min)	+++	+++	+++	+++	++
Health Utilities Index (HUI)	Horsman et al [13]	Interval	15	QOL, general	Self-administered (10 min)	+++	+++	+++	+++	++[f]

[a] Numerical characteristics: interval (continuous number), ordinal (ranking of criteria), or nominal (classification of subjects by number).
[b] Number of responses required in instrument.
[c] Thoroughness: 0, no reported evidence of reliability or validity; +, very basic information only; ++, several types of tests or several studies have reported reliability or validity; +++, all major forms of reliability or validity testing.
[d] Results: 0, no numerical results reported; ?, results unpredictable; +, weak reliability or validity; ++, adequate reliability or validity; +++, excellent reliability or validity.
[e] Sensitivity to change: 0, no results reported; ?, results mixed; +, weak sensitivity to change; ++, adequate sensitivity to change; +++, excellent sensitivity to change.
[f] The Health Utilities Index has only been used in reduction mammaplasty patients.

The senior author (AT) of this article recently published a similar study using the SF-36, MBSRQ, and HUI in 52 breast-reduction patients with a follow-up of 1 year [18]. Mean scores of all measures increased. Additionally, the HUI allows for the calculation of quality-adjusted life years, a means to quantify the benefit of a medical intervention in terms of additional years in perfect health added to a lifespan. In this study, patients gained an estimated 5.32 additional quality-adjusted life years after reduction mammoplasty.

While breast-reduction patients may differ from aesthetic surgery patients in that they have a significant functional impairment, these studies demonstrate that even preference-based outcome instruments are sensitive to change following plastic surgical procedures. It remains to be seen whether significant increases in QOL can be measured after aesthetic surgery.

Summary

In aesthetic surgery, traditional methods of clinical research in measuring outcomes are limited. Outcomes methods may hold great promise for advancing clinical research in aesthetic surgery. Quantification of patient outcome following surgery would allow us to measure the benefit of our interventions. Standardization of outcome assessment would allow for the comparison of techniques. There is a definite need to develop condition-specific instruments in aesthetic surgery. Preference-based QOL instruments will allow for calculation of quality-adjusted life years, economic analysis, and comparisons with other health states. Using outcome methods that have been adopted by other fields of medicine would allow other physicians to understand the benefits of our interventions.

References

[1] Ching S, Thoma A, McCabe R, et al. Measuring outcomes in aesthetic surgery: a comprehensive review of the literature. Plast Reconstr Surg 2003;111(1):469–80.

[2] Clancy CM, Eisenberg JM. Outcomes research: measuring the end results of health care. Science 1998;282:245–6.

[3] Streiner DL, Norman GR. Health measurement scales: a practical guide to their development and use. 2nd edition. New York: Oxford University Press; 1995.

[4] Scientific Advisory Committee of the Medical Outcomes Trust. Assessing health status and quality-of-life instruments: attributes and review criteria. Qual Life Res 2002;11:193–205.

[5] Cash TF. Users' manual for the multidimensional body–self relations questionnaire (3rd revision). 2000. Available at: www.body-images.com. Accessed November 9, 2007.

[6] Guyatt GH, Feeny DH, Patrick DL. Measuring health-related quality of life: basic sciences review. Ann Intern Med 1993;70:225–30.

[7] Cella DF, Tulsky DS. Measuring quality of life today: methodological aspects. Oncology 1990; 5:29–38.

[8] Ware JE. SF-36 health survey: manual and interpretation guide. Boston: The Health Institute, New England Medical Center; 1993.

[9] Harris DL, Carr AT. The Derriford appearance scale (DAS59): a new psychometric scale for the evaluation of patients with disfigurements and aesthetic problems of appearance. Br J Plast Surg 2001;54:216–22.

[10] Anderson RC, Cunningham B, Tafesse E, et al. Validation of the breast evaluation questionnaire for use with breast surgery patients. Plast Reconstr Surg 2006;118(3):597–602.

[11] Kerrigan CL, Collins ED, Kneeland TS, et al. Reliability of a disease-specific, paper-based, self-administered utility instrument for women with breast hypertrophy. Plast Reconstr Surg 2000; 106:280.

[12] The Euroqol Group. EuroQol: a new facility for the measurement of health-related quality of life. The EuroQol Group. Health Policy 1990; 16:199–208.

[13] Horsman J, Furlong B, Feeny D, et al. The health utilities index (HUI): concepts, measurement properties, and applications. Health Qual Life Outcomes 2003;1:54.

[14] Guyatt GH, Naylor CD, Juniper E, et al. Users' guides to the medical literature: XII. How to use articles about health-related quality of life. JAMA 1997;277:1232–7.

[15] Sarwer DB, Wadden TA, Whitaker LA. An investigation of changes in body image following cosmetic surgery. Plast Reconstr Surg 2002;109(1): 363–9.

[16] Bolton MA, Pruzinsky T, Cash TF, et al. Measuring outcomes plastic surgery: body image and quality of life in abdominoplasty patients. Plast Reconstr Surg 2003;112(2):619–25.

[17] Hermans BJE, Boeckx WD, DeLorenzi F, et al. Quality of life after breast reduction. Ann Plast Surg 2005;55(3):227–31.

[18] Thoma A, Sprague S, Veltri K, et al. A prospective study of patients undergoing breast reduction surgery: health-related quality of life and clinical outcomes. Plast Reconstr Surg 2007;102(1): 13–26.

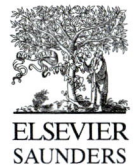

The Role of the Randomized Controlled Trial in Plastic Surgery

Achilleas Thoma, MD, MSc, FRCS(C), FACS[a,b,c,*], Sheila Sprague, MSc[a], Claire Temple, MD, FRCSC[d], Stuart Archibald, MD, FRCSC, FACS[c,e]

- Challenges in the design and execution of RCTs in plastic surgery
  Surgical equipoise
  The surgical learning curve
  Differential care
  Randomization
  Concealment
  Expertise-based study design
- Blinding
  Intention-to-treat analysis
  Limiting loss to follow-up
  Treatment effect and implications to sample size
- Summary
- References

A randomized controlled trial (RCT) is an experiment in which individuals are randomly allocated to receive or not receive an experimental preventative, therapeutic, or diagnostic procedure, and then followed to determine the effect of the intervention [1]. The RCT is generally regarded as the most scientifically rigorous study design to evaluate the effect of a new surgical intervention. This type of study offers the maximum protection against biases in the choice of treatment, as it facilitates blinding and reduces selection bias, and it balances both known and unknown prognostic factors across treatment groups [2,3]. Lack of randomization predisposes a study to potentially important imbalances in baseline characteristics between two study groups.

The importance of randomization is illustrated by a classic example from the neurosurgical literature. In the 1970s and early 1980s, neurosurgeons frequently performed extracranial-intracranial bypass surgeries in which the superficial temporal artery was anastomosed to the middle cerebral artery for stroke prevention. Comparisons of outcomes among nonrandomized cohorts of patients, who for various reasons did or did not undergo this procedure, concluded that the bypass procedure had a salutary outcome on these patients. However, when a large multicenter RCT was undertaken,

---

[a] Department of Clinical Epidemiology and Biostatistics, McMaster University, 293 Wellington Street North, Suite 110, Hamilton, ON L8L 8E7, Canada
[b] Department of Surgery, Division of Plastic Surgery, McMaster University, St. Joseph's Healthcare, 50 Charlton Avenue East, Hamilton, ON L8N 4A6, Canada
[c] Surgical Outcomes Research Centre (SOURCE), McMaster University, St. Joseph's Healthcare, 50 Charlton Avenue East, Hamilton, ON L8N 4A6, Canada
[d] University of Western Ontario, Hand and Upper Limb Centre, St. Joseph's Health Centre, 268 Grosvenor Street, Suite D0-215, London, ON N6A 4L6, Canada
[e] Department of Surgery, Division of Head & Neck Surgery, McMaster University, St. Joseph's Healthcare, 50 Charlton Avenue East, Hamilton, ON L8N 4A6, Canada
* Corresponding author. 206 James Street South, Suite 101, Hamilton, ON L8P 3A9, Canada.
E-mail address: athoma@mcmaster.ca (A. Thoma).

randomly allocating patients to surgical or medical treatment, the study demonstrated surgery increased adverse outcomes in the immediate post-surgical period, but did not decrease stroke over medical management [4].

Observational studies are the common study design in plastic surgery. Unfortunately, this design frequently overestimates the treatment effect, because the physician or patient determined whether a patient received the experimental surgical treatment. For example, imagine a hypothetical observational study in which the investigators compared the deep inferior epigastric perforator (DIEP) flap to the pedicled transverse rectus abdominus myocutaneous (TRAM) flap for breast reconstruction, and found higher rates of success (positive outcomes) with the DIEP flap. This finding could be because investigators chose thin patients to have the DIEP flap, and the heavy patients to undergo the pedicled TRAM flap. This patient selection introduces bias and the beneficial effect may not have anything to do with the choice of the novel technique (ie, DIEP flap). As such, observational studies tend to overestimate the actual treatment effects when compared with data from RCTs [2,5–7].

Research in plastic surgery attempts to determine the impact of novel surgical intervention on such outcomes as control of pain, ability to return to activities of daily living, and ability to return to work. These events are often referred to as the trial's primary and secondary outcome measures. There are a number of factors, however, that can determine the frequency in which the trial's primary and secondary outcomes can occur. These prognostic factors can include the age and sex of the patient, the severity of the condition before the patient entered the study, and current treatment. Diabetes and cardiac conditions are examples of comorbid conditions that can affect the frequency of the trial's target outcomes. Workers compensation status can also affect the return to work target outcome [8].

If a particular study does not take into consideration the known and unknown prognostic factors (ie, the prognostic factors are not balanced in the experimental and control groups), then it is likely the outcomes of the study will be biased. The study will then overestimate or underestimate the true effect of the surgical intervention.

Prognostic factors often influence the surgeon's recommendations and patient's decisions about surgical interventions. For example, in postmastectomy breast reconstruction, the surgeon may recommend a free TRAM flap in an obese patient, but a pedicled TRAM flap in a thin patient, if the surgeon believes these choices are likely to ensure vascular integrity of the flap. As a result, observational studies show larger treatment effects than RCTs [2,5–7]. Only in the properly designed RCT are we certain that there is a balance of known and unknown prognostic factors between the treatment groups, thereby minimizing bias and maximizing the chance that the results are valid.

Although the RCT is considered the most sound research design, or "the most powerful tool in modern clinical research" [9], it is not a panacea to answer all clinical questions. The popular belief that the RCT alone produces trustworthy results, and that all observational studies are misleading, does disservice to patient care, clinical investigation, and the education of health care professionals [10]. In many situations, conducting an RCT is not feasible, necessary, or appropriate. It would not be feasible to perform an RCT to examine very rare events. For instance, it would not be feasible to compare in an RCT the following two deep venous thrombosis prophylaxis approaches for a straightforward abdominoplasty: intermittent lower extremity pump versus subcutaneous heparin, with the outcome being lethal pulmonary embolism. With a rare target event, such as lethal pulmonary embolism, in elective cosmetic surgery, the sample size required would be prohibitively huge (thousands of patients), rendering such a study infeasible.

To examine the deleterious effect of smoking on survival of microvascular flap of the lower extremity, it is not possible to prescribe smoking to one arm of a study. In this hypothetical question of harm, a case-controlled study design is the most appropriate and ethical study design to answer the question (see the article by Sprague, McKay, and Thoma in this issue).

Despite the well-known limitations of the observational design and the strengths of the RCT, plastic surgeons have not embraced the RCT to the same degree as their colleagues from various medical subspecialties. Possible reasons for this could be difficulty accruing enough patients, difficulty perceiving that the question posed is worth answering, inconvenience (for surgeons and patients), and economic disincentive. Furthermore, when RCTs have been conducted in the field of plastic surgery, the validity of these studies is often in question because of poor methodology. The mere reporting of a surgical study as "randomized" does not infer validity; one should exercise caution before rushing to adopt the study's findings [11].

Thoma and colleagues reviewed all of the RCTs that compared endoscopic carpal tunnel release (ECTR) to open carpal tunnel release (OCTR) and found methodologic flaws in the reporting of those studies [12]. These RCTs also gave conflicting conclusions. If these RCTs had been properly powered and conducted, they would have converged around a common estimate of effect. When reporting is flawed, it is also possible that the methodology may have been inexact, casting serious doubts on the validity of these studies.

In order to conduct high quality, large RCTs, to produce an estimated effect with a narrow confidence interval, multicenter collaboration is required. The research culture in plastic surgery needs to adopt this initiative. Participation in multicenter research initiatives is our responsibility, as our surgical activities frequently performed are expensive for society. In light of limited health care resources, there is an opportunity cost in performing surgical procedures, which are less effective than alternatives (see the article by Thoma, Strumas, Rockwell, and McKnight in this issue). Plastic surgery journals are replete with alternative choices, in a seeming competition of who will invent another technique to solve a surgical problem. If there is one truly effective technique, we have been misallocating society's scarce resources in choosing the suboptimal techniques. It behooves all of us to collaborate in order to definitively answer clinically important questions in the field of plastic surgery.

Challenges in the design and execution of RCTs in plastic surgery

The execution of a plastic surgery RCT is challenging. This section discusses these challenges and some strategies to ameliorate them. Topics covered include: surgical equipoise, surgical learning curve, differential care, randomization, concealment, expertise-based design, blinding, intention-to-treat analysis, loss to follow-up, and treatment effects and implications for sample size calculations.

Surgical equipoise

A precondition to undertaking an RCT is the existence of the state of equipoise. Equipoise reflects a state of genuine uncertainty about the benefits or harms that may result from each of two or more regimens [13]. A state of equipoise is an indication for an RCT, because there are no scientific or ethical concerns about one regimen being better for a particular patient [13–15].

It would be unwise to perform an RCT comparing two plastic surgical procedures (A and B) to treat a particular problem if plastic surgeons truly believed that treatment A is superior. The only justification for performing an RCT is the state of ambivalence between A and B, and controversy amongst experts with some professing that one is better. Beyond surgical equipoise, the controversial "novel" procedure needs to be commonly performed and resource intensive to justify the energy and costs of an RCT.

Examples in plastic surgery where recent research has identified equipoise despite a number of small RCTs, is the unsolved controversy between ECTR and OCTR [16,17] and the numerous arthroplasty techniques of the carpo-metacarpal joint of the thumb [18]. The multiple cutaneous flaps used for head and neck reconstruction would also satisfy the precondition for equipoise, as it is unclear that one flap is superior to another (ie, free osseocutaneous radial forearm versus free fibular flap). As microsurgical reconstructions of the head and neck are complex, lengthy procedures that consume a lot of health care resources, an RCT would be appropriate to compare techniques. In the field of melanoma, the issue of whether sentinel lymph node biopsy and directed lympaedenectomy improves survival beyond wide excision alone, was another example of equipoise, before the results of the RCT conducted by the Multicenter Selective Lymphadenectomy Trial (MSLT) Group was published in 2006 [19]. This RCT randomized patients to wide excision and observation of regional lymph nodes, with lymphadenectomy in case of nodal relapse, or to wide excision and sentinel node biopsy, with immediate lymphadenectomy if the sentinel node was positive. Among patients with nodal metastases, the 5-year survival was higher amongst those who underwent immediate lympadenectomy, as directed by sentinel node biopsy, than those who required therapeutic lymphadenectomy once regional metastases became clinically evident.

The surgical learning curve

When a new drug is compared to a standard drug or placebo, there is no technical skill requirement to administer the different pills. In contradistinction, in comparing a "novel" to the "usual" intervention in plastic surgery, the learning curve of the novel surgical technique becomes an important issue, especially in some procedures, such as ECTR. An endoscopic technique differs in approach and instrumentation. Likewise, the DIEP is more complex and challenging than the pedicled TRAM flap in postmastectomy reconstruction.

Surgeons have a learning curve for all procedures. The learning curve refers to the surgeon's cumulative experience in performing a new intervention in which there is continuous refinement of patient selection, operative technique, and postoperative care [11]. For sentinel lymph node biopsy, the MSLT group has determined that completion of 55 procedures is required to reliably reduce nodal relapse [19]. When a surgical RCT shows that Approach B is superior, surgeons who previously preferred A, question whether the surgeons in the RCT had the appropriate skill level with Approach A [20]. If the surgeons in the randomized controlled trial were not equally proficient with the approaches before the randomized controlled trial is begun, the results could be misleading [20]. It is inappropriate to compare familiar to unfamiliar surgical procedures, because mistakes and adverse events are more likely to occur with the unfamiliar procedure, and the results will be biased against the novel technique [21–23].

Consider the DIEP versus the free TRAM debate in postmastectomy reconstruction. An investigator may have been performing the free TRAM flap reconstruction for the first 15 years of his/her career and now wishes to compare resource costs between the TRAM and the DIEP flap (the novel intervention) in an RCT. If he or she does not master the learning curve for the DIEP flap first, the costs may appear to be higher for the wrong reasons. He or she may have more failing DIEP flaps and more return cases to the operating room for emergency revisions, and he or she may be slower in the operating room in harvesting the DIEP flap, increasing operating room utilization costs. The investigator will conclude that the DIEP flap is an inferior procedure to the free TRAM flap, as the operating room time was longer and more re-explorations required more operating room visits.

For this reason, readers gain confidence when the trial reports that the surgeons had demonstrated completion of the learning curve before starting the study (ie, the study reports all surgeons completed a prerequisite number of cases with the procedures under evaluation before starting the RCT) [24]. An RCT should only be considered when the participating surgeons are equally capable of performing the novel and the comparator interventions. For example, in comparing the vertical scar to the inferior pedicle technique in breast reduction (Clinical Trials Number NCT00149344, www.clinicaltrials.gov), all participating surgeons were required to watch videotape detailing each step of the vertical scar technique (the novel procedure). Each surgeon had to then perform 10 cases using the vertical scar breast reduction, complication-free, before contributing cases to the RCT. Failure to control for the learning curve may underestimate the effect size of the novel intervention.

Differential care

In pharmaceutical studies, an investigator can conceal the experimental pill from the placebo pill until the end of the study. In plastic surgery, blinding usually disappears once the incision is made. A plastic surgeon who participates in an RCT may inadvertently bias the results while the patient is in the operating room, or during follow-up encounters by providing a little extra care, such as improving hemostasis, excluding house staff from elements of the procedure, or increasing the frequency of follow-up for the technique toward which he or she may be biased. Additionally, the surgical intervention may include additional procedures that may influence the postoperative results and overestimate the effect size. If the surgeon was biased towards the vertical scar technique for breast reduction, the outcome could be biased in favor of this technique by performing additional liposuction on the fullness of the anterior axillary fold and the lateral chest wall only with this technique, and not the inferior pedicle technique. Providing preoperative antibiotics to the vertical scar technique patients would also bias the results toward this technique.

Differential care is a real threat to the study and is best avoided by standardizing the procedure as much as possible (ie, using procedure manuals). In the breast reduction RCT, alluded to above, all the surgeons involved, participated in the preparation of a procedure manual for each of the two competing interventions. The manual prohibited the use of liposuction or any other procedure not listed. Besides ensuring that all participating surgeons agree on how the procedure should be performed before the trial begins, other methods of standardizing the surgical procedures include holding teaching sessions prior to the trial, auditing surgical performance throughout the trial, and stratifying patients by surgeon at the time of randomization [25]. Stratifying by surgeon will not eliminate the variation in how a procedure is performed, but it will reduce the imbalance between groups [26]. Investigators should detail how the surgical protocol was standardized in their final report.

In addition to standardizing the protocol for the different surgical techniques, it is necessary to standardize the nonsurgical portion of the patients' care, including pre- and postoperative treatment, medications, physiotherapy, and frequency of follow up. The MSLT group standardized follow-up to three per month for years 1 and 2, four per month for year 3, six per month for year 4 and 5, and yearly thereafter until 10 years. In this manner, patients randomized to sentinel lymph node biopsy and patients randomized to observation would each be followed at identical intervals [19].

Randomization

The methods of randomization frequently are poorly described in published RCTs [27,28]. Even more worrisome, the crucial step of randomization is often performed using a faulty method, which invalidates the entire study. In a recent systematic review of the RCTs that compared the ECTR versus OCTR, Thoma and colleagues [12] found that

73% of the studies used faulty or inadequate method of randomization. The method of randomization is so crucial to the validity of the study that it needs to be done correctly and be transparent. Using even or odd birth years or an alternate chart number are inadequately concealed and are prone to selection bias [6]. The use of random number tables or computer programs to generate the sequences are correct ways to randomize patients.

The gold standard in randomization is an automated telephone or internet randomization system [1]. In Morton and colleagues' [19] trial, randomization was done centrally, in a stratified fashion, and in random permuted blocks of four, six, and eight patients. Stratification factors included Breslow thickness (1.20 mm to 1.79 mm versus 1.80 mm to 2.50 mm) and extremity versus other site. A 60 to 40 ratio of biopsy to observation was used. Table 1 of Morton and colleagues' article [19] shows the baseline characteristics of the patients in the observation and biopsy arms, with no difference for all known prognostic factors. One assumes that all unknown prognostic factors are balanced as well based on their sound method of randomization. In the RCT comparing the vertical scar versus inferior pedicle technique for breast reduction, the randomization of treatment allocation occurs 30 minutes before surgery while the patient is in the operating waiting area. The plastic surgeon calls the preprogrammed automated system that randomizes the patient to either the vertical scar technique or the inferior pedicle technique. Once the patient is allocated to a treatment arm, the surgeon marks the pattern on the patient's breasts. In this manner, selection bias is avoided.

Concealment

The comparison of a novel to a prevailing plastic surgical technique is different from the comparison of medications. When comparing medications, the size, color and taste of competing pills can be standardized to conceal the treatment allocation from all parties; in surgical trials this blinding is not possible.

To ensure concealment of the treatment allocation, those who are making the decision about patient eligibility are not aware of the arm of the study to which a particular patient will be allocated (ie, vertical scar versus inferior pedicle technique). If the treatment allocation is not concealed, an investigator may enroll patients with more severe, or alternatively milder, conditions, which may bias the results of a trial [3,29]. For example, if the investigator believed that the vertical scar technique is superior, and the treatment arm could be previewed by using semitransparent envelopes which carried the allocation (after the randomization was performed), the investigator could selectively enroll patients with a low body mass index (BMI) (less than 25 kg/m^2) to the vertical scar technique, and those with high BMI to the inferior pedicle technique. Selectively excluding some of the eligible patients, because of prior knowledge of the group to which they would be allocated if they participated in the study, introduces selection bias [26]. In using even or odd birth year or chart number, investigators may consciously or subconsciously select patients to enter the study based on knowledge of the group to which they will be allocated. Using opaque sealed envelopes helps conceal patient allocation; however, even in these instances investigators have previewed envelope codes using a bright light or by steaming the envelope open [26]. The authors' preference is an automated internet or telephone randomization system at the coordinating center.

Expertise-based study design

Because it takes training and experience to develop expertise in surgical interventions, individual surgeons tend to apply a single surgical approach to treat a specific problem [30]. The restricted expertise that results can compromise the validity of a conventional RCT [30]. One solution is the expertise-based study design, in which patients are randomized to surgeons who do their operation of preference, as opposed to randomizing patients to a treatment group. This ensures that the surgeons in the RCT have experience with the intervention they are doing [24]. One caveat is that each participating center must have some surgeons doing each type of operation to limit institutional factors (postoperative nursing care) impacting on the outcome [20]. Therefore, a balance of surgeons doing the study interventions at each clinical site allows readers more confidence that the results are related to the surgical interventions and not to institutional factors [20].

The increased use of the expertise-based design will enhance the validity, applicability, feasibility, and ethical integrity of RCTs in surgery [30]. Expertise-based RCTs may have greater applicability and feasibility than conventional trials in many surgical subspecialties [30]. This design is useful to examine the efficacy of novel, technically demanding procedures, such as the use of supermicrosurgery in raising periumbilical perforarator flaps above the rectus fascia. These flaps require using 11-0 nylon sutures to complete 0.4 mm anastomoses [31]. One drawback to the expertise design is that these procedures are not technically generalizable to a community hospital or even to some academic centers. Another drawback of the expertise design is that it adds cost and increases complexity of the randomization, as it requires stratification by surgeon and center. For these reasons, the authors advocate that the majority of clinically important problems in plastic surgery can be solved by the traditional RCT and do not require the expertise-based design.

Blinding

The concept of blinding is frequently misunderstood. Though some claim the lack of blinding as a cause of invalidation of a study, this may not be the case. Ideally one should ask first: was blinding possible? If it was possible, why wasn't it done?

In many pharmaceutical studies, blinding is relatively easy. In surgery, however, this is not possible, at least at present. Perhaps in the future, using preprogrammed robots, blinding of the surgeon will be possible. The terms "single," "double," or "triple" blinded can be misleading unless the investigators indicate exactly who was blinded. There are six potential levels of blinding: (1) the patients, (2) the clinicians who administer the treatment, (3) the clinicians who care for the patients during the trial, (4) the individuals who assess the patients throughout the trial and collect the data, (5) the data analyst, and (6) the investigators who interpret and write the results of the trial [26].

In the breast reduction RCT, the surgeons performing the surgery could not be blinded, nor could the patients, as they could see the shape of the scar (ie, a "lollipop" versus "anchor" shaped scar). However, the biostatistician who will analyze the data at the completion of the study was able to be blinded. Therefore, this RCT would be considered single blinded. If one of the outcomes was comparison of postoperative pain during hospitalization, covering both breasts with dressings and concealing the scar could blind the patient. This RCT would be considered double blinded (biostatistician and patient).

In pharmaceutical trials, the investigators, the patients, and the assessors of the outcome can all be blinded, as the placebo may look, smell, and taste exactly like the investigated pill. In plastic surgical trials, the surgeons cannot be blinded because they know which surgical technique they performed. In addition, the patients usually know which technique they received based on the shape of the suture line and eventual scar. If a patient knows they received the experimental treatment and the patient believes the novel therapy is better than the traditional technique, the patient may feel better than those who receive the traditional treatment, even if the there is no underlying difference between the two methods. This observation has been called "the placebo effect" [32]. The same holds true for the plastic surgeon or nurse who is the designated assessor for the study. Even if the two surgical groups have been kept prognostically balanced, if the assessors are not blinded, the study can still be biased.

Without blinding of the assessor, one surgical arm may receive more frequent or thorough measurement of outcome or cointervention. Additional physiotherapy, positive interpretation of marginal findings, or differential encouragement during performance tests, are all pitfalls of inadequate blinding [33]. The results will be swayed in favor of the surgical group that received additional attention. In the MLST study, the patients, surgeons and assessors knew the members of the experimental arm, as these patients would have had a scar over the regional lymph node basin [19].

One solution is to keep the scar concealed from the assessor. Where the scars are similar, this concealment is not an issue, unless the assessor has access to the operative report. For example, the scars are identical in studies of carpal tunnel release, with or without synovectomy, and of various arthroplasty techniques of the carpo-metacarpal joint of the thumb [18]. Even if scars are identical, the assessor may have access to the patient's operative note and is not truly blinded. This is the norm when conducting studies in a small surgical practice with limited support staff, where research nurses access the patient's chart to complete the case report forms.

In most RCTs in plastic surgery, it is possible to blind the data analyst and the investigators who interpret and write the results of the RCT. In the melanoma study, it was not mentioned whether the data analyst was blinded. Ideally, the investigators should consider these issues prior to embarking on the study.

Intention-to-treat analysis

Intention-to-treat analysis is a concept that causes consternation among surgeons whenever it rears its head at journal clubs or scientific meetings. It is therefore important to explain it. Randomization can only accomplish the goal of balancing groups, with respect to both known and unknown determinants of outcomes, if patients are analyzed in the groups to which they are randomized [34]. Randomization may be corrupted if not all patients receive their assigned surgery.

Imagine, for example, the scenario where the next patient was assigned to undergo the inferior pedicle technique for breast reduction. As the surgeon prepares to make the incision, he or she notices a scar in the inferior pole of the breast not previously noted. The surgeon worries about performing the inferior pedicle technique (the one assigned) because of fear of devascularising the nipple, so he or she changes plans and carries out the vertical scar technique (not assigned). Should this patient be analyzed in the group in which the computerized automated system assigned her (ie, inferior pedicle) or the group in which she received the surgery (ie, vertical scar)?

If plastic surgeons include poorly destined patients in one surgical treatment group and not the other, then even a suboptimal surgical procedure may appear to be effective. Intention-to-treat analysis avoids this potential bias [34]. The analysis of the outcomes is based on the treatment arm to which patients were randomized, and not on which surgical treatment they received. The intention to treat analysis includes all patients, regardless of whether they actually satisfied the entry criteria, received the treatment to which they were randomly allocated, or deviated from the protocol. Analyzing patients based upon the treatment they actually receive can upset the prognostic balance of randomization because the reasons why patients who do not take their medication or do not receive a particular surgical intervention are often related to prognosis [35]. With intention-to-treat analysis, all the known and unknown prognostic factors will be equally distributed in the two surgical groups [11].

Of the 1,347 patients enrolled in the MLST trial, 58 patients did not receive their assigned care, 22 patients assigned to nodal observation underwent sentinel node biopsy, and 36 patients assigned to sentinel node biopsy underwent observation. The entire group of 1,327 (20 patients withdrew before treatment) patients was analyzed according to the intention-to-treat principal, and the remaining 1,269 patients who received the assigned treatment were analyzed separately. In this study, the results were consistent regardless of the method of analysis [19].

Limiting loss to follow-up

Failure to account for all patients at end of the study may invalidate the RCT [11]. An incomplete follow-up biases the results of a trial when patients who drop out are different from those for whom follow-up is complete. This is exaggerated further when there are differential dropout rates between study groups [36]. It is imperative to achieve a high rate of patient follow-up to minimize the chance that this type of bias will affect the results of an RCT in plastic surgery.

Some patients who are lost to follow-up may have had a bad outcome or died. Alternatively, some patients may have had an excellent outcome and did not bother to return for follow-up appointments [11]. Researchers suggest that fewer than 5% loss probably leads to little bias, whereas greater than 20% loss potentially threatens validity [37,38]. In Morton's trial, 4.3% of the observation arm and 4.6% of the sentinel node biopsy patients were lost to follow-up, which could be considered a negligible loss [19]. Chronic versus acute surgery, the outcome event rates, and the length of the follow-up all influence loss to follow-up rates [37]. A large loss to follow-up rate can reduce the study power.

The occurrence of the event of interest among patients is uncertain after a specified time when follow-up data collection ends. It is unknown when or whether the event of interest occurred subsequently. Such patients are described as censored [13,39,40]. These patients still contribute to the study up to the time at which their outcome status was last known. The censoring effect requires the use of appropriate analytic methods, such as survival analysis [40,41].

Sprague and colleagues [36] suggest a number of strategies for reducing loss to follow-up in surgical RCTs (see Box 1). Research staff needs to be highly organized, to allocate time for contacting patients who are at risk of becoming lost to follow-up, and to be committed to the study. This attention to detail requires a substantial amount of time, increased personnel resources, and consequently, funding [36]. Many surgical trials have been conducted with limited funding, which contributes to the loss to follow-up [42].

In the melanoma trial, the sample size was adjusted at the second of four planned interim analyses. The initial sample size calculation estimated that 900 patients would be required for a type I error rate of 5%, and a power of 90%. However, the early experience of the patients entering the trial was a lower risk for recurrence or death, hence fewer events than expected. At this juncture, the sample size was increased to 1,200 patients given the paucity of events. All told, 1,347 patients were enrolled to balance accrual among study centers, and to include all patients who had signed consent before the enrollment was closed [19].

Treatment effect and implications to sample size

One common mistake in plastic surgery RCTs is the choice of sample size [43]. Investigators often arbitrarily choose a convenient sample size from their practice. The usual finding is that there is no difference between the experimental and the standard technique. If an underlying effect truly exists, but went unnoticed because of an underpowered study, this is termed a "type II error." A study with a small sample size can only identify a statistically significant difference if the expected effect size is large. For example, the effect size between the competing techniques ECTR versus OCTR is small. Although a small effect difference may appear of no consequence, when a procedure is common it

> **Box 1: Primary, secondary, and tertiary strategies for reducing loss to follow-up [36]**
>
> *Primary strategies: trial design*
> - Exclude individuals who are unlikely to complete follow-up (ie, patients with no fixed address, those who report a plan to move out of town in the next year, those who are intellectually challenged without adequate family support, those who are uncertain about their willingness to complete follow-up)
> - Fully inform patients of the burden of the study prior to randomization
> - Provide patients with information on their injuries, the risk of complications, potential treatment effects, expectations for personal benefit from study participation, and motivation for adherence with follow-up visits and research protocols
> - At the time of randomization, obtain contact information for the patient, primary care physician, and alternate contacts
> - Prior to hospital discharge, have the attending surgeon take time with the patient to emphasize how the study will help future patients who have the same problem, and to discuss the importance of returning for all follow-up visits
> - Design the study's follow-up schedule to coincide with normal surgical follow-up visits
> - Have study staff at the methods center contact the clinical sites regularly to discuss and to help locate any patients with overdue visits
>
> *Secondary strategies: innovative designs to minimize losses*
> - Schedule follow-up appointment times around patient preferences
> - Provide patients with reminders for upcoming follow-up visits, maintain regular contact, and obtain information on any planned change in residence
> - Minimize the amount of time patients spend waiting at a follow-up visit and encourage patients to complete questionnaires while waiting
> - Reduce the demands of participation in the study by following for patients who have a language barrier, cognitive impairment, or as a last resort for patients who do not want to complete the quality of questionnaires by following for primary events only.
> - Closely monitor data for missed and overdue follow-up visits
> - Have methods center staff develop strategies with the clinical staff to locate patients with overdue follow-up appointments
> - Contact patients or alternate contacts by telephone for follow-up, even during evenings and weekends if necessary
>
> *Tertiary strategies: locating patients who are labeled lost to follow-up*
> - If the methods center receives an early withdrawal form, have methods center staff contact the clinical center immediately to discuss the patient's situation.
> - If a patient finds it difficult to continue, study staff negotiates with the patient to encourage them to continue with the study and may offer to reduce the demands of study participation
> - Continue trying to contact lost patients and all alternate contacts until you are able to reach someone to determine the patient's status, unless the telephone lines have been disconnected.
> - Have clinical staff watch for patients reappearing in their clinic for other reasons
> - Have staff at the methods center help the clinical centers contact patients they are having a difficult time reaching
>
> *From* Sprague S, Leece P, Bhandari M, et al, on behalf of the SPRINT investigators. Limiting loss to follow up in a multi-centre randomized controlled trial in orthopaedic surgery. Control Clin Trials 2003;24:723; with permission.

is clinically relevant and carries important economic consequences. When the effect size is expected to be small or moderate, the investigators need to estimate the baseline risk of the outcome event in the control group, and estimate an expected relative risk reduction in order to calculate the sample size [43]. In many instances, the sample size will be in the thousands, rather than the usual sample of hundreds. The inadequacy of the sample size in a recent meta-analysis of RCTs that compared ECTR and OCTR was recently reported [17].

Summary

If the field of plastic surgery is to advance, it has to adopt well-established methodologic principles from clinical trialists and epidemiologists. Small underpowered RCTs are unlikely to provide the answers needed. They confuse, rather than clarify the issue; they conclude that there is no difference between surgical procedures, whereas in fact there may be a true difference (type II error). On the other hand, small studies also capitalize on the play of chance in that they may factitiously identify a difference (type I error) [43]. Consulting a biostatistician is helpful to perform a sample size calculation before embarking on an RCT and will determine what sample size is required to show whether a true difference exists [43].

Traditionally plastic surgeons have worked and published in solitary or small group fashion. Rarely do they see large multicenter trials. Recent evidence suggests that the sample size required in carrying out the definitive study for the authors' example, ECTR versus OCTR (in which the effect size is very small), requires the recruitment of some 5,000 patients [44]. To conduct such a "mega randomized controlled trial" requires collaboration, as well as resources far beyond the means of a few surgeons. Society support, such as the American Society of Plastic Surgeons and the Canadian Society of Plastic Surgeons, is necessary, as is collaboration with biostatisticians, health economists, epidemiologists, and clinical trialists.

Finally, the mere fact that an article carries in its title the words "randomized controlled trial" does not confer to it validity. Not all published RCTs are of good methodologic quality. Guidelines exist for the appraisal of their methodologic quality [11,45]. Only RCTs of high methodologic quality should be seriously considered.

In conclusion, the RCT is considered to be the strongest clinical study design for its ability to reduce bias and balance prognostic factors. However, there are several situations where the RCT is inappropriate or not the best study design to address the research question. Not all of the questions faced in plastic surgery can be answered by the RCT design, such as in cases where the end points are rare (feasibility issues) and in cases where harmful outcomes are considered (ethical considerations). While RCTs in plastic surgery continue to be rare, there remain many clinically important questions in this specialty that could be best addressed with a randomized design. Small RCTs are inadequately powered to provide the answers we are seeking. To conduct high-quality, large RCTs, multicenter collaboration is required. The research culture in plastic surgery requires change; only participation in multicenter initiatives will answer many of the clinical problems in our specialty.

References

[1] Guyatt G, Rennie D. Users' Guides to the Medical Literature: A Manual for Evidence-Based Clinical practice. In: Guyatt G, Rennie D, editors. JAMA & Archives Journals. Chicago: American Medical Association; 2002.
[2] Coditz GA, Miller JN, Mosteller F. How study design affects outcomes in comparisons of therapy. I Med. Stat Med 1989;8:441–54.
[3] Schultz KF, Chalmers I, Hayes RJ, et al. Empirical evidence of bias: Dimensions of methodological quality associated with estimates of treatment effects in controlled trials. JAMA 1995;273: 408–12.
[4] Haynes RB, Mukherjee J, Sackett DL, et al. Functional status changes following medical or surgical treatment for cerebral ischemia: results in the EC/IC Bypass Study. JAMA 1987; 257:2043–6.
[5] Sacks HS, Chalmers TC, Smith H Jr. Sensitivity and specificity of clinical trials: randomized v historical controls. Arch Intern Med 1983;143:753–5.
[6] Chalmers TC, Celano P, Sacks HS, et al. Bias in treatment assignment in controlled clinical trials. N Engl J Med 1983;309:1358–61.
[7] Emerson JD, Burdick E, Hoaglin DC, et al. An empirical study of the possible relation of treatment differences to quality scores in controlled randomized clinical trials. Control Clin Trials 1990;11:339–52.
[8] Ayeni O, Thoma A, Haines T, et al. Analysis of the reporting of return to work in studies comparing open and endoscopic carpal tunnel release: a review of randomized controlled trials. Can J Plast Surg 2005;13:117–79.
[9] Silverman WA. Gnosis and random allotment. Control Clin Trials 1981;2:161–4.
[10] Concato J, Shah N, Howitz RI. Randomized controlled trials, observational studies, and hierarchy of research designs. N Engl J Med 2000; 342:1887–92.
[11] Thoma A, Farrokhyar F, Bhandari M, et al. For the Evidence-Based Surgery Working Group. Users' Guide to the Surgical Literature. How to assess a randomized controlled trial in surgery. Can J Surg 2004;47:200–8.
[12] Thoma A, Chew TC, Veltri K. Application of the CONSORT statement to randomized controlled trials comparing endoscopic carpal tunnel release (ECTR) and open carpal tunnel release (OCTR). Abstracts of American Association for Hand Surgery Annual Meeting 2004 Palm Springs, California. Presented on 16 Jan 2004.
[13] Last MJ. A dictionary of epidemilogy. 3rd Edition. New York: Oxford University Press; 1995.
[14] Schafer A. The ethics of the randomized clinical trial. N Engl J Med 1982;307:719–24.
[15] Pocock SJ. Ethical issues. In: Clinical trials. Toronto: John Wiley & Sons; 1984. Chapter 7. p. 100–109 [Reprinted 1993].
[16] Thoma A, Veltri K, Haines T, et al. A systematic review of reviews comparing endoscopic and open carpal tunnel decompression. Plast Reconstr Surg 2004;113:1184–91.
[17] Thoma A, Veltri K, Haines T, et al. A meta-analysis of randomized controlled trials comparing endoscopic and open carpal tunnel decompression. Plast Reconstr Surg 2004;114(5):1137–46.
[18] Martou G, Veltri K, Thoma A. Surgical treatment of osteoarthritis (OA) of thecarpometacarpal

(CMC) joint of the thumb: a systematic review. Plast Reconstr Surg 2004;114(2):421–32.
[19] Morton DL, Thompson JF, Cochran AJ, et al. Sentinel-node biopsy or nodal observation in melanoma. N Engl J Med 2006;355(13):1307–17.
[20] Devereaux PJ, McKee M, Yusif S. Methodological issues in surgical randomized controlled trials. Clin Orthop Rel Res 2003;413:25–32.
[21] Bonenkamp JJ, Songun I, Hermans I, et al. Randomized comparison of morbidity and mortality after DI and D2 dissection for gastric cancer in Dutch patients. Lancet 1995;345:745–8.
[22] Ramsay CR, Grant AM, Wallace SA, et al. Statistical assessment of the learning curves of health technologies. Health Technol Assess 2001;5:1–79.
[23] Mohammed MA, Cheng KK, Rouse A, et al. Bristol, Shipman, and clinical governance. Shewhart's forgotten lessons. Lancet 2001;357:463–7.
[24] McCulloch P, Taylor I, Sassako M, et al. Randomized trials in surgery: problems and possible solutions. BMJ 2002;321:1448–51.
[25] McLeod RS. Issues in surgical randomized trials. World J Surg 1999;23:1210–4.
[26] Jadad A. Randomized Controlled Trials. London: BMJ Books; 1998.
[27] Altman DG, Dore CJ. Randomization and baseline comparisons in clinical trials. Lancet 1990;335:149–53.
[28] Moher D, Fortin P, Jadad AR, et al. Completeness of reporting of trials in languages other than English: implications for the conduct and reporting of systematic reviews. Lancet 1996;347:363–6.
[29] Moher D, Pham B, Jones A, et al. Does the quality of reports of randomized trials effect estimates of intervention efficacy reported in meta-analyses? Lancet 1998;352:609–13.
[30] Devereaux PJ, Bhandari M, Clarke M, et al. Need for expertise based randomised controlled trials. BMJ 2005;330:88.
[31] Koshima I, Inagawa K, Yamamoto M, et al. New microsurgical breast reconstruction using free paraumbilical perforator adiposal flaps. Plast Reconstr Surg 2000;106:61–5.
[32] Kaptchuk TJ. Powerful placebo: the dark side of the randomized controlled trial. Lancet 1998;351:1722–5.
[33] Guyatt GH, Pugsley SO, Sullivan MJ, et al. Effect of encouragement on walking test performance. Thorax 1984;39:818–22.
[34] Hollis S, Campbell F. What is meant by intention to treat analysis? Survey of published randomized controlled trials. Br Med J 1999;319:670–4.
[35] Bhandari M, Guyatt GH, Swiontowski MF. Users' Guide to the Orthopaedic Literature: How to use an article about a surgical therapy. J Bone Joint Surg 2001;83A:916–26.
[36] Sprague S, Leece P, Bhandari M, et al. on behalf of the SPRINT investigators. Limiting loss to follow up in a multi-centre randomized controlled trial in orthopaedic surgery. Control Clin Trials 2003;24:719–23.
[37] Schultz KF, Grimes DA. Sample size slippages in randomised trials: exclusions and the lost and wayward. Lancet 2002;359:781–5.
[38] Sackett DL, Richardson WS, Rosenberg W, et al. Evidence-based medicine: How to practice and teach EBM. New York: Churchill Livingstone; 1997.
[39] Harrell FE Jr. Regression Modeling Strategies, with application to Linear Models, Logistic Regression, and Survival Analysis. New York: Springer-Verlag; 2001. p.49.
[40] Elwood M. Critical appraisal of Epidemiological Studies and Clinical Trials. New York: Oxford University Press, Inc.; 1998. p. 43.
[41] Armitage P, Berry G. Statistical Methods in Medical Research. London: Blackwell Scientific Publications; 1994. p. 469.
[42] Solomon MJ, McLeod RS. Surgery and the randomized controlled trial: past, present, and future. Med J Aust 1998;169:380–3.
[43] Caddedu M, Haines T, Forrkhyar F, et al. Users' Guide to the Surgical Literature: How to assess power and sample size. Can J Surg, in press.
[44] Thoma A, Haines T, Goldsmith C, et al. Design of a randomized controlled trial comparing endoscopic carpal tunnel release (ECTR) and open carpal tunnel release (OCTR): Canadian collaborative initiative. Can J Plast Surg 2003;11:96.
[45] Thoma A, Chew R, Sprague S, et al. Application of the CONSORT statement to randomized controlled trials comparing endoscopic and open carpal tunnel release. Can J Plast Surg 2006;14(4):205–10.

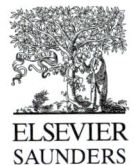

The Use of Cost-effectiveness Analysis in Plastic Surgery Clinical Research

Achilleas Thoma, MD, MSc, FRCS(C), FACS[a,b,c,*], Nick Strumas, MD, FRCSC[b], Gloria Rockwell, MD, MSc, FRCSC[d], Leslie McKnight, MSc[b]

- Preconditions for cost-effectiveness analysis
    - Identification of all relevant treatment options
    - Perspective taken
    - The costs and consequences of the competing interventions
- Cost-effectiveness
- Types of economic evaluations
- Discounting costs
- Methodologic considerations
- Sensitivity analysis
- Controversy using incremental cost-utility ratios
- Use of economic evaluations in clinical practice
- Summary
- References

Over the past 2 decades, there have been pressures to control health care spending in many jurisdictions. The term, "cost effective," increasingly is in common parlance. In 1993, the United States Public Health Service convened a Panel on Cost-effectiveness in Health and Medicine. One of the mandates of the panel was to reach a consensus on how to perform cost-effectiveness analysis (CEA) and help those performing such studies to improve their quality and encourage their comparability [1].

This article reviews the principles underpinning economic evaluations and how they can be applied to plastic surgery. Illustrative examples are drawn from economic evaluations published by the authors.

Plastic surgery as a specialty is prolific in the introduction of new techniques, procedures, and approaches to solving specific problems. For example, in autologous breast reconstruction, there are various techniques to create a new breast. Considering just one donor flap site, such as the abdomen, there are several flaps that can be used, including the pedicled transverse rectus abdominis myocutaneous (TRAM) flap, free TRAM flap, deep inferior epigastric perforator (DIEP), muscle sparing TRAM flap, and superficial inferior epigastric artery (SIEA). Every time one of these flaps is used, resources are used, in terms of personnel, equipment, facilities, and time. The choice of using one

[a] Department of Clinical Epidemiology and Biostatistics, McMaster University, Hamilton Health Sciences Centre, 1200 Main Street West, Hamilton, ON L8N 3Z5, Canada
[b] Department of Surgery, Division of Plastic Surgery, McMaster University, St. Joseph's Healthcare, 50 Charlton Avenue East, Hamilton, ON L8N 4B6, Canada
[c] Surgical Outcomes Research Centre (SOURCE), McMaster University, St. Joseph's Healthcare, 50 Charlton Avenue East, Hamilton, ON L8N 4A6, Canada
[d] Department of Surgery, Division of Plastic Surgery, University of Ottawa, 401-1919 Riverside Drive, Ottawa, ON K1H 1A2, Canada
* Corresponding author. 206 James Street South, Suite 101, Hamilton, ON L8P 3A9, Canada
E-mail address: athoma@mcmaster.ca (A. Thoma).

technique over another is made most commonly using " a hunch," "surgical intuition," or "previous experience." On rare occasions, the decision may be based on scientific evidence, which regrettably often is based on a lower level of evidence (see the article by Sprague, McKay, and Thoma in this issue).

The term, cost effective, frequently is used in the surgical literature to justify the introduction of a new procedure. The term often is used, however, inappropriately. The investigators may have performed a direct medical cost comparison between two successful competing interventions and if the novel procedure is less costly, they label it as cost effective. When considering costs, however, all the resources consumed by the novel procedure should be considered. The value of all these resources is the lost opportunity to use them in another way.

When comparing novel versus usual surgery techniques, cost is only one component of the analysis. Researchers fail to consider that the outcomes (effectiveness) may be different. Outcomes are mortality, morbidity (in terms of short-, intermediate-, and long-term complications), and patient satisfaction. The probabilities of these outcomes may be different between the competing interventions. To label a novel intervention as cost-effective, a proper economic evaluation must be performed comparing the alternative courses of action in terms of costs and consequences between the two competing interventions.

Preconditions for cost-effectiveness analysis

Health care resources are scarce and it behooves everyone to use them judiciously. The economic evaluation of newly introduced surgical procedures is necessary to ensure using those procedures that produce the best outcomes for the resources consumed. An economic evaluation helps when considering and comparing a "new" technique to a "standard" or prevailing technique.

The three preconditions for performing an economic evaluation comparing surgical interventions are:

1. Identification of all relevant treatment options or surgical techniques to solve the problem
2. Identification of the perspective (viewpoint) taken for the study
3. Measurement of the costs and consequences of the novel and prevailing technique as accurately as possible

Identification of all relevant treatment options

The first precondition for an economic evaluation is identifying systematically all the relevant treatment options or surgical techniques to solve a problem. For example, in breast reconstruction, when a decision is made to use only tissue from the abdomen, surgeons must be familiar with all the options from pedicled TRAM to SIEA. Abdominal autologous tissue is not the only available technique for breast reconstruction, and a comparison to other techniques, such as tissue expander/implants or latissimus dorsi or gluteal flaps, should be considered.

Perspective taken

The second precondition for an economic evaluation is identifying clearly the viewpoint taken in the economic evaluation. There are several viewpoints that can be considered, based on who is benefiting from the new intervention. Is it the patient, hospital, third-party payer (eg, workers' compensation board, Medicare, health maintenance organizations, ministry of health, or national health service), or society? The perspective taken depends on the research question being pursued (see the article by Thoma, McKnight, McKay, and Haines in this issue).

The benefits obtained from an intervention are not the same across all possible beneficiaries. For example, comparing the use of implants and DIEP in breast reconstruction, from a ministry of health's perspective (viewpoint), the use of the implants may be preferable as the use of resources up front is much less. The operating room (OR) time used for implants is only a fraction of the time required for a DIEP, and patients may be discharged home the same day as compared with a possible hospitalization of from 4 to 8 days for a DIEP. From a patient's perspective, however, the use of implants may not provide the best outcome, as symmetry of the breasts may not be achieved because of the possibility of downstream complications associated with the implant, such as failure, capsular contracture, and malposition. It is mandatory, therefore, in any clinical research that compares novel to prevailing technologies, to be explicit about who is benefiting from the procedure. Still better, consider multiple perspectives. For example, in an ongoing randomized controlled trial (RCT) comparing the vertical scar to the inferior pedicle technique in breast reduction, the authors are piggy-backing on an economic evaluation. The decision was made a priori to consider three separate perspectives: the patients', the Ministry of Health's, and society's (Clinical Trials Number NCT00149344, www.clinicaltrials.gov).

The costs and consequences of the competing interventions

The third precondition for an economic evaluation is ensuring an effort is made to measure the costs and consequences as accurately as possible not only of the novel or new technique or approach but also of the standard technique (it is also possible that new techniques can be compared with no intervention). The real value of novel surgical techniques is not only the cost (resources used) but also the value of the benefits achievable in some other area of health care delivery (eg, another surgical technique) that has been forgone by committing more scarce resources to the novel surgical technique. With a limited pool of health care resources, when one hand takes more from the pool, the other has to give something up, and the impact of this is defined in health economics as opportunity cost.

Cost calculation can be divided into three main categories: (1) direct costs, which can be variable (as costs increase, outputs increase) or fixed (stable costs, such as overhead); (2) indirect costs, which usually represent productivity losses resulting from morbidity (eg, loss of wages resulting from inability to work) or, rarely, mortality; and (3) intangible costs, which are those represented by nonfinancial considerations, such as pain, grief, and suffering.

When calculating costs in a clinical study, costs and charges have to be differentiated. Charges for surgical procedures are substantially different from costs. For example, what patients pay to a hospital for breast reconstruction usually is higher than the actual costs to perform surgery. This discrepancy is more problematic in the United States, where many hospitals work on a profit business model, as compared with the Canadian publicly funded health care system, where there is only one third-party payer (the government). In a recent study, Taira and colleagues [2] compared four methods of estimating costs in three separate trials involving percutaneous coronary revascularization: (1) hospital charges; (2) hospital charges converted to costs by use of hospital-level cost-to-charge ratios; (3) hospital charges converted to costs by use of department-level cost-to-charge ratios; and (4) itemized laboratory costs with nonprocedural hospital costs generated from department-level cost-to-charge ratios. The investigators found that although there were big differences in the magnitude of the estimates obtained by the various methods, the method used to approximate costs did not affect the main results of the economic comparisons of any of the trials. They also concluded that conversion of hospital charges to costs on the basis of department-level cost-to-charge ratios seems to represent a reasonable compromise between accuracy and ease of implementation [2].

When reporting the results of an economic analysis, it is important for investigators to tabulate the quantity of resources used in their natural units rather than summarizing the costs. For example, in an RCT comparing two techniques of breast reduction, the authors intend to report the mean OR time it takes to complete each procedure and the mean hospitalization in days. In this way, other investigators in other geographic jurisdictions can take the resource use from this study and plug in their costs/units of resource used and see if the novel procedure is cost effective in their setting.

Economic evaluations in plastic surgery consider the costs in terms of resource use and consequences (short and long term) of surgical interventions. They also consider the decisions made by surgeons and the impact these choices have on the health of the patients and that of other patients who are in need of the same scarce health care resources. In plastic surgery, the authors make the choice to use a surgical technique based on many criteria, some explicit (evidence based) but more often implicit (ie, what works in our hands). Economic evaluations can help guide the decision-making process.

Cost-effectiveness

In clinical practice, the outcomes (consequences) of procedures frequently are considered but the costs involved seldom are. It is important to change the surgical paradigm under which surgeons have been trained and currently are practicing. Surgeons are, to a great degree, custodians of the health care system, which has limited resources. Changing the paradigm in which surgeons are working, Fig. 1 suggests that every time surgeons perform procedure "A" they should reflect not only on the consequences (clinical outcomes) of procedure A but also the costs associated with this choice compared to those of alternative surgery "B" [3]. When two surgical techniques are compared, for example DIEP and free TRAM for breast reconstruction, there are nine possible outcomes based on incremental cost and effectiveness of one procedure over another (Fig. 2) [4]. Some decisions are clear-cut; for instance, cell 1 of Fig. 2 represents a case where the novel procedure is less costly and more effective than the traditional technique, a win-win situation. In this situation, the novel technique should be used. Similarly, if a procedure falls into cell 2, more expensive and less effective, it should be rejected. Many decisions, however, are not as straightforward. Most new surgical procedures fall into cell 7: they are more effective but also more expensive. Here is a dilemma. Should the novel procedure be used or rejected? In such cases, given the constraints of limited health care resources, economic analyses can facilitate decision making [5,6].

Another way of representing these concepts is the cost-effectiveness plane (Fig. 3) [4]. If a new

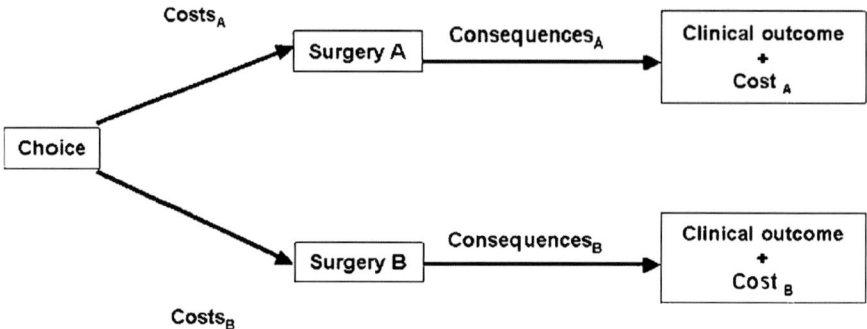

Fig. 1. Comparative analysis of competing surgical interventions. For every surgical decision made, consider not only the consequences (clinical outcomes) but also the costs of both interventions.

surgical intervention falls in the right lower quadrant, there is a win-win scenario, as the new intervention is less expensive and more effective. If it falls in the left upper quadrant, it is rejected, as it costs more and is less effective, a lose-lose scenario. Most new procedures fall in the right upper quadrant (more costly and more effective). This situation corresponds to cell 7 in Fig. 2. It is here that economic analysis facilitates decision making as to using or rejecting a new intervention.

Types of economic evaluations

There are four types of economic evaluations commonly discussed in the literature (features described in Table 1): (1) cost analysis: a cost comparison study, not a full economic evaluation; (2) CEA; (3) cost-utility analysis (CUA); and (4) cost-benefit analysis (CBA). In the initial design phase of an economic evaluation, the eventual type of analysis (cost analysis, CEA, or CUA) may not been known unless the effectiveness of both treatments already is established in the literature. For instance, if the clinical outcomes of the competing interventions are the same (eg, successful replantations with similar probabilities of success and failures), then the study is simplified to a cost analysis or cost-comparison study. In this situation, the less costly yet equally effective treatment option should be considered.

If differences in effectiveness between the two techniques are identified in the course of a study, the study can be designated as CEA, CUA, or CBA, depending on how the consequences (outcomes) are measured. If natural units are used (eg, lives saved or successful replants), the economic analysis is labeled CEA. If the outcomes are quality-adjusted life years (QALYs), the study is labeled CUA. If the outcomes are measured in dollars or pounds, the study is labeled CBA.

In a CEA, the health outcomes are reported in natural units, such as lives saved, replants saved, or successful breast reconstructions. The results of the study are reported, for instance, as $40,000 per leg saved if comparing two orthopedic

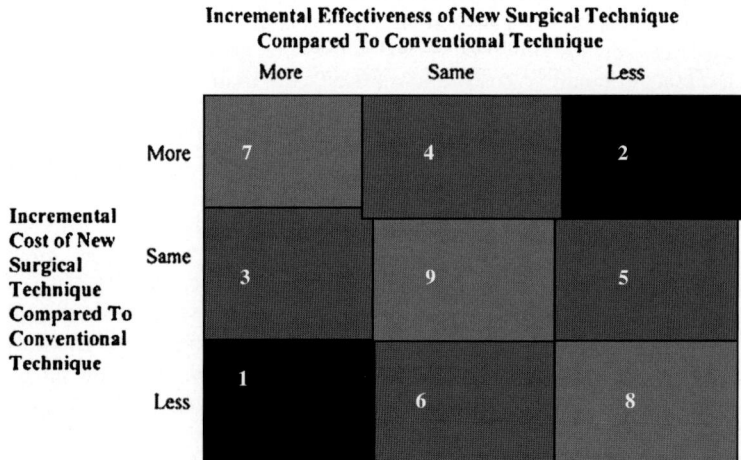

Fig. 2. Nine possible outcomes when comparing a new surgical technique and a conventional surgical technique. (From Thoma A, Sprague S, Tandan V. Users guide to the surgical literature: how to use an article on economic analysis. Can J Surg 2001;44:347; with permission.)

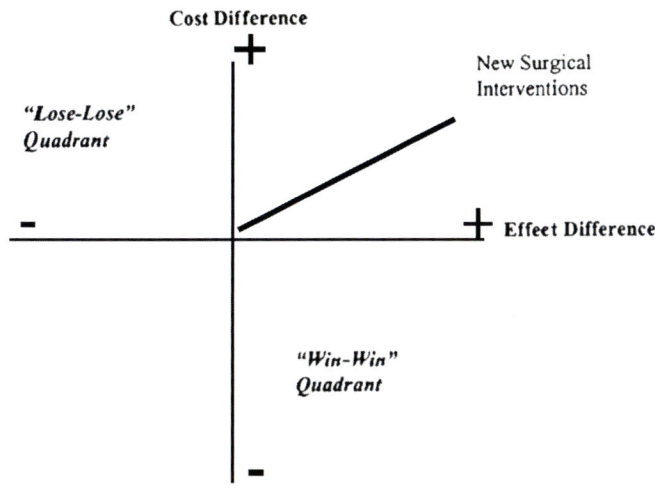

Fig. 3. Cost-effectiveness plane. (From Thoma A, Veltri K, Khuthaila D, et al. Comparison of the deep inferior epigastric perforator (DIEP) and free transverse rectus abdominis myocutaneous (TRAM) flap in post-mastectomy reconstruction: a cost-effectiveness analysis. Plast Reconstr Surg 2004;113:1650–61; with permission.)

approaches to treating compound fractures of the tibia. The problem with this type of analysis is that it is difficult to compare disparate surgical interventions, which can have important but different clinical outcomes. Imagine that Medicare announces that it will reimburse those novel procedures in which a CEA is performed within a limited budget. Suppose that the American Society of Plastic Surgeons undertook such a study and compared the "supramicrosugery" transfer of a periumbilical

Table 1: Distinguishing characteristics of the four main economic evaluations (cost analysis, cost-effectiveness analysis, cost-utility analysis, and cost-benefit analysis)

Type of analysis	Valuation of costs	Identification of outcomes (consequences)	Metric used in the analysis
Cost analysis	Monetary units (eg, dollars or pounds)	None	None. This analysis is only a comparison of costs.
Cost-effectiveness analysis	Monetary units (eg, dollars or pounds)	Common effect of interest. Common outcomes to the competing surgical interventions but with different degrees of success (eg, successful flaps, successful replants, lives saved, sick days averted, or hospital days averted).	Dollars per natural unit (eg, dollars per successful replant, dollars per life saved, or dollars per hospital day averted)
Cost-utility analysis	Monetary units (eg, dollars or pounds)	Single or multiple effects that not necessarily are common to both interventions. Outcomes are measured in utilities that are transformed to QALYs.	Dollars per QALY or pounds per QALY
Cost-benefit analysis	Monetary units (eg, dollars or pounds)	Single or multiple effects not necessarily common to both surgical procedures and calculated in dollars or pounds	Monetary units (eg, dollars or pounds)

flap (new procedure) to a DIEP flap for breast reconstruction, finding that this new procedure would cost $40,000 per successful breast reconstruction. The American Orthopedic Association does its own economic evaluation, however, comparing two types of knee replacements. They find that the novel technique costs $50,000 per successful knee replacement. How are the bureaucrats in Medicare going to decide which new procedure to use if there is funding to use only one of these two novel technologies? Does the $40,000 per successful breast reconstruction confer more value to the society than the $50,000 per successful knee replacement or vice versa?

CEA is used best when trying to determine the allocation of resources within a given field. As in the example discussed previously, it is difficult to compare interventions with different health outcomes using a CEA. In addition, there may be more than one outcome of interest for a given intervention. Surgeons might want to know not only how much longer a person may live, but also the quality of life a patient might have after an intervention. CEA is unable to address this. Lastly, some outcomes may be more valued than others and this needs to be considered. Again, CEA is unable to do this.

CUA can help address many of these concerns. CUA and CEA are similar on the cost side. In a CUA, however, the outcome of a surgical procedure is measured in terms of utility (a measure of preference for a particular health state). Utilities (preferences) are transformed into QALYs. The results are expressed as cost per QALY gained [4]. This outcome measure incorporates changes in quantity of life (eg, reduction of mortality) and quality of life (eg, reduction in morbidity) into a standard metric.

The CUA is a variant of CEA and is encountered commonly in studies originating in the United Kingdom and Canada [7,8]. In the United States, CUA and CEA are used interchangeably. The advantage of a CUA is that by using a common metric for effectiveness, QALYs, disparate procedures whose outcomes are completely different from the ones encountered in plastic surgery can be compared.

QALYs are derived from utilities. A utility is the preference or desirability for a health outcome. Utilities can be obtained from quality-of-life assessment instruments, including visual analog scales, generic scales (eg, Health Utilities Index Mark 2-3, Quality of Well-Being, Short Form 6D, and EuroQol), the standard gamble, and time tradeoff. Utility scales are defined such that perfect health and death are assigned values of 1 and 0, respectively [3].

The standard gamble presents participants with a hypothetical scenario, consisting of choices A and B [9]. Choice A consists of varying probabilities of successful surgery, for example, composite facial allotransplantation (defined as successful surgery and no subsequent complications) and associated complications (including death), and choice B represents their current health state (for example, facial disfigurement). Participants are asked to estimate to the largest percentage risk for complications (or death) they would be willing to accept to be relieved of their current health state (eg, remaining in facial disfigurement) [9].

With the Time Trade Off (TTO), participants also are presented with the same hypothetical scenario of two choices [9]. Choice A is associated with a shortened life expectancy of "x" years resulting from immunosupression after composite facial allotransplantation, and choice B with a given life expectancy of "t" years. In other words, patients are asked about how much of their life expectancy they are willing to trade off to avoid the health state denoted by choice B (for example, facial disfigurement). The utility value of the health state in question is estimated by the proportion between the shortened life expectancy (x) and the full life expectancy of the intermediate outcome (t) [9].

The CUA probably is the most useful type of analysis in a prospective study comparing two competing interventions. When a CUA is done parallel to a methodologically sound RCT, it provides the best evidence available to guide the decision-making process. (For those interested in learning the nuances of performing a CUA parallel to an RCT in plastic surgery, see the recent article by Thoma and colleagues [10]).

CBA attaches a monetary value to the consequence of an intervention. CBA has its grounding in welfare economics and is based on the principle of consumer sovereignty—individuals are the best judges of their own welfare. Although a CEA or CUA can inform on the cost of achieving a particular goal (incremental cost of life year gained, a case of disease detected, and so forth), it cannot indicate whether or not the goal is worth achieving given opportunity costs. That is, it does not answer the question as to which goods and services consumers are willing to give up to have the new program [11]. CEA and CUA avoid monetary valuation of health outcomes as part of their analysis; however, administrative decision makers ultimately have to place a monetary value on an outcome to facilitate comparisons between the disparate uses of the health care budget, which is allocated in terms of dollars, not resources. Cost benefit analysis already has this aspect built into it [3]. In performing a CBA, a willingness-to-pay

(WTP) approach can be used. WTP can be determined directly or indirectly. Indirect methods infer values from actual decisions individuals make. Contingent valuation is an example of a direct technique. It uses survey questions to determine how much individuals are willing to pay for the good or service in question. It is useful in the absence of free markets, such as in the case of health care, by presenting consumers with a hypothetical market that allows them to buy the goods or services in question. WTP becomes appealing because of the following [12]:

1. Benefits are measured in the same units as costs. This permits the net benefit (benefit minus cost) of a program to be calculated.
2. WTP allows for intersectoral comparisons (eg, transportation versus health care versus education).
3. WTP allows tradeoffs between health and other goods.
4. WTP can capture externalities (eg, WTP for a vaccination for other for fear we get infected ourselves).
5. WTP is a sensitive measure of outcome.
6. WTP can be modified to capture the unique nature of health as a good.

There are criticisms of WTP, including the hypothetical nature of the WTP question. Another concern is WTP does not address equity. WTP may be influenced by income distribution and the ability to pay. Therefore, there is some resistance to adopting CBA in health care. Whether or not this is acceptable must be weighed against the benefits the WTP model brings. (For those interested in more detailed explanations of WTP and CBA, more advanced sources are recommended [3].)

Discounting costs

The costs and benefits of a surgical intervention or health care program may not occur at the same time point. For example, implant-based reconstructions may require future operations, to correct capsular contractures, deflation, or mechanical failure of the implants, or rebalancing procedures to the contralateral breast. These future costs and benefits need to be considered in an economic evaluation, because their costs in the future will not be the same as their costs today. Discounting is the process of determining the present value of the costs and benefits experienced in future. It is based on a time preference that society prefers to experience benefits now and pay later (even if there were no interest rates or inflation). Therefore, discounting places a higher value on current costs and benefits than those experienced in the uncertain future; 5% per annum is the rate used commonly.

Methodologic considerations

Economic evaluations can be divided into two methodologic types. The first type, called a deterministic analysis, is one in which primary data are lacking. The second type of evaluation is one in which there are primary data and is called a stochastic analysis (these two types are explained in detail later).

To illustrate a deterministic analysis, a published economic analysis is used as an example [13]. Thoma and colleagues performed an economic analysis comparing the DIEP to the free TRAM flap in breast reconstruction. They performed a CEA to determine if the DIEP was a cost-effective procedure from the viewpoint of the Ministry of Health from the Province of Ontario in Canada. A decision analytic model was used (Fig. 4). A decision analytic model is "a quantitative clinical epidemiology tool for physicians (and patients) who wish to quantify expected risks, benefits, utilities and sometimes costs associated with alternative treatment options for individual patients" [14]. A decision analytic tree was constructed to illustrate the health state possibilities for the DIEP and free TRAM flap (Fig. 5). The costs of the competing interventions easily were obtained from the Canadian health care system, which was the only payer for the procedures. The various direct costs were identified, including surgeons' and anesthetists' fees and the OR and hospitalization costs. To calculate the actual OR and hospital costs, the investigators performed a thorough literature search to identify the OR time for the competing interventions and the mean hospital stay. They multiplied the OR time by the cost per hour in a university hospital and the per diem cost of hospitalization to find the true hospital cost (Table 2).

To identify the clinically important consequences of the two competing interventions, Thoma and colleagues undertook a review of the plastic surgery literature. The seven most common complications identified, labeled "health states," were used in the analysis (see Fig. 5). By pooling the results, the probability of each important health state occurring with each technique (for example, hernia repair is 0.04 for the DIEP) was obtained [13]. These probabilities are shown in Fig. 5. The outcomes (consequences: successful surgery and complications) were measured in utilities (preferences) using the "feeling thermometer" technique, a visual analog scale [15]. These utilities were transformed into QALYs using the following formula:

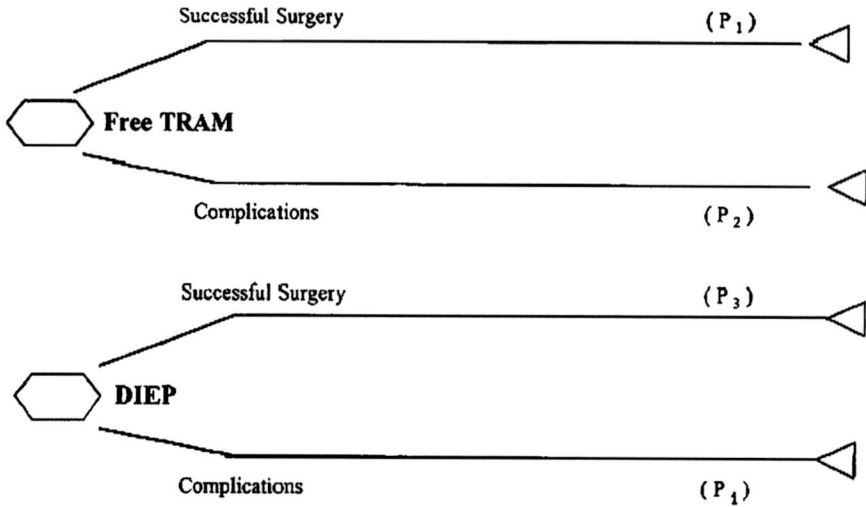

Fig. 4. Decision analytic tree illustrating the possible health state probabilities of the DIEP and free TRAM flaps. P_1–P_4 are the probabilities of successful outcomes or complications for the competing interventions. (*From* Thoma A, Veltri K, Khuthaila D, et al. Comparison of the deep inferior epigastric perforator (DIEP) and free transverse rectus abdominis myocutaneous (TRAM) flap in post-mastectomy reconstruction: a cost-effectiveness analysis. Plast Reconstr Surg 2004;113:1650–61; with permission.)

QALY = (duration of health state)
× (utiliy of health state)
+ (future remaining life expectancy-duration of health state)
× (utility of successful reconstruction)

A deterministic analysis calculates the expected-costs and expected QALYs of each branch of the decision analytic tree. To obtain these expected values, the investigators multiplied the costs and QALYs by the probability of each pathway (Table 3). The investigators then calculated the incremental cost-utility ratio (ICUR), which determines if the novel procedure is cost effective. The ICUR represents the marginal cost per marginal unit of utility and is calculated as follows:

ICUR = $\Delta C / \Delta U$
= (mean $\text{cost}_{\text{DIEP}}$ − mean $\text{cost}_{\text{freeTRAMflap}}$) / (mean $\text{QALY}_{\text{DIEP}}$ − mean $\text{QALY}_{\text{freeTRAMflap}}$)

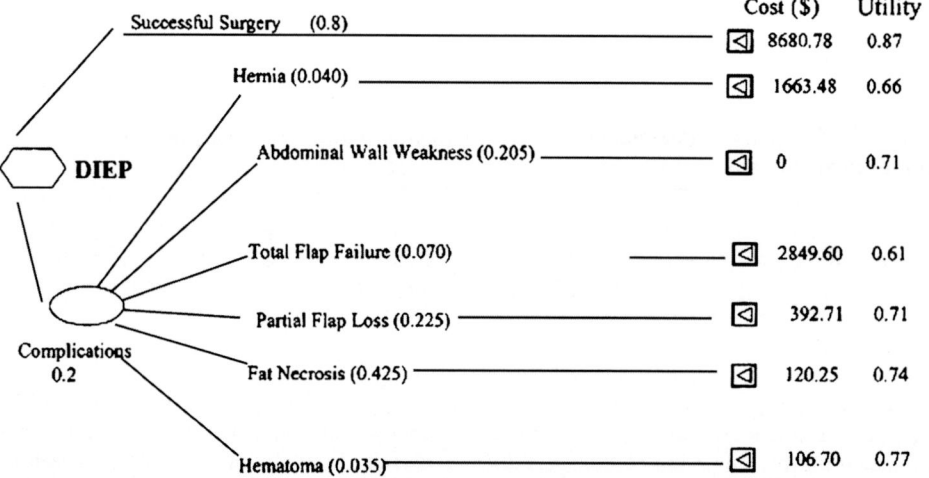

Fig. 5. Decision analytic tree illustrating probabilities (shown in parenthesis), costs, and utilities of each health state for the DIEP. A similar decision analytic tree was constructed for the free TRAM (not shown here). (*From* Thoma A, Veltri K, Khuthaila D, et al. Comparison of the deep inferior epigastric perforator (DIEP) and free transverse rectus abdominis myocutaneous (TRAM) flap in post-mastectomy reconstruction: a cost-effectiveness analysis. Plast Reconstr Surg 2004;113:1650–61; with permission.)

Table 2: Estimated costs (in Canadian dollars for Province of Ontario, Canada)

	Free TRAM flap	DIEP flap
Surgeon	$2204.82	$2204.82
Anesthesia	$1024.00	$776.82
OR + hospital	$6797.69	$5699.14
Total direct cost	$10,026.52	$8680.79

From Thoma A, Veltri K, Khuthaila D, et al. Comparison of the deep inferior epigastric perforator (DIEP) and free transverse rectus abdominis myocutaneous (TRAM) flap in post-mastectomy reconstruction: a cost-effectiveness analysis. Plast Reconstr Surg 2004;113:1650–61; with permission.

This ratio, which integrates costs and effectiveness, indicates whether or not to adopt the novel procedure. The result is represented as cost per QALY. In simple words, it relays how much it costs to prolong the life of a patient by 1 extra year in perfect health. The higher the ICUR, the greater the incremental cost for an additional healthy year of life. The investigators found the ICUR to be $1464.30 per QALY. This result means that prolonging the life of a patient for 1 year in perfect health would cost society $1464.30. It generally is accepted that if an intervention has an ICUR below the threshold of $20,000 per QALY, there is a strong indication for its acceptance. Alternatively, if the ICUR is above the threshold of $100,000 per QALY, there is an indication for its rejection [16]. According to these guidelines, the DIEP was considered a cost-effective procedure when compared with the free TRAM flap.

There is much discussion in the literature regarding the interpretation and application of the ICUR. In particular, the quantitative thresholds proposed by Laupacis and colleagues in 1992 [16] are criticized for being arbitrary and outdated, although they remain in frequent use [17–19]. For example, the National Institute for Health and Clinical Excellence of the British National Health Service uses £20,000 per QALY as their ICUR threshold for acceptance of new technologies [20,21].

In a stochastic analysis, primary outcome data is obtained directly from patients. Additionally, costs (direct and indirect) are obtained from the same patients. From this data, means and standard deviations can be calculated. This is the ideal type of analysis. For example, in a pilot study, Thoma and colleagues (2004) performed a stochastic analysis comparing two techniques of carpal tunnel release [9]. In one technique, the carpal ligament was transected in the classical manner. In the other technique, the ligament was incised in a Z-plasty fashion and then sutured to itself. The intention was to release it but still preserve it. A previous publication claimed that the latter technique is a superior method to dealing with the carpal tunnel syndrome [22]. In this pilot study, the utilities were calculated as quality-adjusted weeks (a fraction of QALYs), as the time horizon for the study was 6 weeks, when the majority of patients resumed their activities of daily living or returned to work. The ICUR showed that this novel procedure not only produced less effectiveness at 6 weeks but also was more expensive. The procedure fell into the lose-lose quadrant of the cost-effectiveness plane, providing evidence to reject this novel technique.

Another example of a stochastic study is the ongoing RCT comparing the vertical scar technique to the inferior pedicle technique for breast reduction (Clinical Trials Number NCT00149344, www.clinicaltrials.gov). Parallel to the RCT, health care resource use (eg, operating times or length of hospital stay), out-of-pocket expenses by patients and caregivers, and patients' return to work are recorded

Table 3: Utilities, costs (in Canadian dollars), and quality-adjusted life years for free transverse rectus abdominis myocutaneous

Health state	Utility	Cost ($)	Expected cost ($)	Quality-adjusted life year	Expected quality-adjusted life year
Successful surgery	0.87	10,026.52	6336.76	29.23	18.47
Total flap failure	0.61	2849.60	45.09	20.50	0.32
Hernia	0.66	1663.48	89.99	29.17	1.58
Abdominal wall weakness	0.71	0	0	23.86	2.46
Partial flap loss	0.71	392.71	19.22	29.20	1.43
Fat necrosis	0.74	120.25	14.56	29.20	3.54
Hematoma	0.77	106.70	2.67	29.22	0.73

A similar table was constructed for the DIEP flap (not shown here).
From Thoma A, Veltri K, Khuthaila D, et al. Comparison of the deep inferior epigastric perforator (DIEP) and free transverse rectus abdominis myocutaneous (TRAM) flap in post-mastectomy reconstruction: a cost-effectiveness analysis. Plast Reconstr Surg 2004;113:1650–61; with permission.

for the year after the breast reduction surgery. Patients are provided with diaries to record their use of health care (eg, family doctor and emergency room visits) and any related out-of-pocket expenses (eg, medication expenses). Health care use and out-of-pocket expenses are recorded at each follow-up visit (1, 6, and 12 months after surgery). The effectiveness in this clinical trial is measured in QALYs gained with each technique. At the completion of the trial, the costs and QALYs will be computed and entered into the ICUR formula. This calculation will indicate if the vertical scar technique is cost effective or not.

Sensitivity analysis

When performing economic evaluations, there can be uncertainties in estimating costs and utilities if they are not measured directly from a study population (as in deterministic studies) or if broad confidence intervals around the means exist (as in stochastic studies). A sensitivity analysis is required when uncertainty exists as a means of assessing the robustness of the results when corrections for uncertainty are made—that is, knowing the best case and the worse case scenario results. These corrections can be performed by adjusting the cost, utility, or probability of one variable at a time (one-way sensitivity analysis) or by varying multiple variables at the same time (two-way or multiway analysis). If the final concluding results after the sensitivity analysis still fall within the same quadrant of the cost-effective plane (see Fig. 3) and below an acceptable threshold, it can be concluded that the results are considered robust and believable [4]. Returning to the example of the deterministic analysis study comparing DIEP to the free TRAM flap in postmastectomy reconstruction, a one-way sensitivity analysis was performed to determine if the baseline ICUR calculation of $1464.30 per QALY was robust. In the sensitivity analysis, the probabilities of health state occurrences were assumed identical in the DIEP and the free TRAM flap. When the probability of the health state hernia for DIEP was adjusted to be the same as the probability of hernia for free TRAM flap, the ICUR changed to $1434 per QALY. Similarly, when the probability of flap failure was equal for DIEP and free TRAM flap, the ICUR changed to $1384 per QALY. These results were consistent with the baseline ICUR of $1464.30 per QALY, making the baseline ICUR result believable.

In the RCT comparing the vertical scar and the inferior pedicle technique (discussed previously), because primary data will be available, means and standard deviations of costs and QALYs can be calculated. The sensitivity analysis in this case may take the form, for instance, of recalculating the ICUR by assuming that the costs may be one standard deviation above the mean, whereas the QALYs (effectiveness) may be one standard deviation below the mean for the novel technique to address the issue of uncertainty. The sensitivity analysis will determine the robustness of the point estimate.

Controversy using incremental cost-utility ratios

The threshold ICUR of $20,000 per QALY as a guide to adopting new interventions recently has been challenged; because resources are scarce and we, as surgeons are operating within a fixed budget, all the new procedures whose ICUR is less than $20,000 per QALY cannot be implemented. If they were, it would lead to uncontrolled growth of health care spending. For a fixed budget, a necessary condition for implementing a new intervention that costs more but improves outcome is to identify an existing intervention (or combination of interventions) that if cancelled generates the additional resources necessary for the new intervention [22]. Therefore, the next step after the economic analysis is to identify interventions for cancellation that can fund the new intervention [23].

Use of economic evaluations in clinical practice

The introduction of new techniques in plastic surgery is appealing to surgeons and patients. The claimed superiority of new techniques, however, often is misleading and, at worst, erroneous. If the principles of evidence-based surgery are applied to clinical practice and research, the inclusion of economic evaluations needs to be considered seriously in clinical investigations. One such example that helped the authors alter the way they practice is the use of prophylactic plating of the donor radius after harvesting free radial osteocutaneous flap. A recent CEA [24] showed that prophylactic plating was less effective and more costly than not prophylatic plating, falling into the lose-lose quadrant of the cost-effectiveness plane. With this evidence, the authors abandoned the practice of plating every donor radius prophylactically, freeing resources for other treatments.

In summary, economic evaluations require the following steps:

1. Deciding which treatment groups to compare (new technique versus standard of care).
2. Deciding on timeline of study and using discounting if future expenditures are anticipated.

3. Deciding on economic perspective to take: patient's, Medicare, ministry of health's, national health service's, society's, and so forth.
4. Deciding what to measure as costs (direct or indirect) and consequences (single outcome state or quality of life).
5. Using sensitivity analysis to check for robustness of the conclusions when uncertainty exists.
6. Remembering that there is a fixed pool of health care resources and that decisions of whether or not to adopt a new technique that is more costly and effective depend on the opportunity costs of health care foregone to free resources for the new technique.

Not all economic evaluations appearing in surgery are of high methodologic quality. For the "users" of clinical research, guidelines exist in the appraisal of articles that purport to be economic evaluations in surgery [4]. The authors recommend strongly that the "doers" of clinical research adopt the correct methodology or obtain the help of a health economist before embarking on an economic analysis comparing plastic surgical interventions.

Summary

An economic analysis helps the users and doers of clinical research to identify the best available evidence, which can be applied to patient care. Clinicians tend to consider the outcomes of surgical procedures with little regard for the cost. In an era of diminishing health care resources, there is a need to be accountable for resource use, and this requires determining the cost effectiveness of any new technique compared with the current standard of care. The problem is that most new techniques prove more effective and more costly. CUA is the best study design to inform on whether or not a new technique is cost effective, as it integrates costs and effectiveness, but the effectiveness is measured in a standard metric, QALYs. This type of study is not performed commonly in plastic surgery possibly because of the unfamiliarity of plastic surgeons with the field of health economics and health research methodology. The authors believe that CUA is extremely important and should be incorporated into surgical clinical research.

References

[1] Gold MR, Siegel JE, Russell LB, et al. Cost-effectiveness in heath and medicine. Oxford University Press; 1996.
[2] Taira DA, Seto TB, Seigrist R, et al. Comparison of analytic approaches for the economic evaluation of new technologies alongside multicenter clinical trials. Am Heart J 2003;145: 452–8.
[3] Drummond MF, Sculpher MJ, Torrance GW, et al. Methods for the economic evaluation of health care programmes. 3rd edition. New York: Oxford University Press; 2005.
[4] Thoma A, Sprague S, Tandan V. Users guide to the surgical literature: how to use an article on economic analysis. Can J Surg 2001;44:347–54.
[5] Russell LB, Gold MR, Siegel JE, et al. The role of cost-effectiveness analysis in health and medicine: panel on cost-effectiveness in health and medicine. J Am Med Assoc 1996;276:1172.
[6] Koshima I, Inagawa K, Yamamoto M, et al. New microsurgical breast reconstruction using free paraumbilical perforator adiposal flaps. Plast Reconstr Surg 2000;106:61.
[7] Sinclair JC, Torrance GW, Boyle MH, et al. Evaluation of neonatal-intensive-care program. N Engl J Med 1981;305:489–94.
[8] Kaplan RM. Health outcome models for policy analysis. Health Psychol 1989;8:723–35.
[9] Cugno S, Sprague S, Duku E, et al. Composite tissue allotransplantation of the face: decision analysis model. Canadian Journal of Plastic Surgery 2007;15(3):145–52.
[10] Thoma A, Veltri K, Haines T, et al. A methodological guide to performing a cost-utility study comparing surgical techniques. Can J Plast Surg 2004;12:179–87.
[11] O'Brien BJ. Assessing the value of a new pharmaceutical: a feasibility study of contingent valuation in managed care. Med Care 1998;36(3):370–84.
[12] O'Brien BJ, Gafni A. When do the "dollars" make sense? Toward a conceptual framework for contingent valuation studies in health care. Med Decis Making 1996;16:288–99.
[13] Drummond MF, Richardson WS, O'Brien BJ, et al. Users' guide to the medical literature. XIII. How to use an article on economic analysis of clinical practice. A. Are the results of the study valid? Evidence-Based Medicine Working Group. J Am Med Assoc 1997;277:1552–7.
[14] Thoma A, Veltri K, Khuthaila D, et al. Comparison of the deep inferior epigastric perforator (DIEP) and free transverse rectus abdominis myocutaneous (TRAM) flap in post-mastectomy reconstruction: a cost-effectiveness analysis. Plast Reconstr Surg 2004;113:1650.
[15] Drummond MF, O'Brien BJ, Stoddart GL, et al. Methods for the economic evaluation of health care programmes. 2nd edition. New York: Oxford University Press; 1997.
[16] Laupacis A, Feeny D, Detsky AS, et al. How attractive does a technology have to be to warrant adoption and utilization? Tentative guidelines for using clinical and economic evaluations. Can Med Assoc J 1992;146:473–81.
[17] Asim O, Petrou S. Valuing a QALY: review of current controversies. Expert Review of Pharmacoeconomics & Outcomes Research 2005;5:667–9.

[18] McGregor M, Caro JJ. QALYs: are they helpful to decision makers? Pharmacoeconomics 2006;24: 947–52.
[19] Vijan S. Should we abandon QALYs as a resource allocation tool? Pharmacoeconomics 2006;24:953–4.
[20] Pearson SD, Rawlins MD. Quality, innovation, and value for money: NICE and the British National Health Service. J Am Med Assoc 2005; 294:2618–22.
[21] Buxton MJ. Economic evaluation and decision making in the UK. Pharmacoeconomics 2006; 24:1133–42.
[22] Jakab E, Ganos D, Cook FW. Transverse carpal ligament reconstruction in surgery for carpal tunnel syndrome. A new technique. J Hand Surg (Am) 1991;16:202–6.
[23] Gafni A, Birch S. Inclusion of drugs in provincial drug benefit programs: should "reasonable decisions" lead to uncontrolled growth in expenditures? CMAJ 2003;168(7):849–51.
[24] Rockwell G, Thoma A. Should the donor radius be plated prophylactically after harvest of a radial-forearm osteocutaneous flap? J Reconstr Microsurg 2004;20:297.

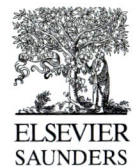

Testing Quality Improvement Interventions

Frank Papanikolaou, MD, FRCSC[a], Charlie H. Goldsmith, BSc, MSc, PhD[b],*

- One hundred thousand lives
- Five million lives
- Safer health care now
- How to perform quality improvement clinical research
- FOCUS-PDCA
- PICOT
- What can surgeons do?
- Benchmarking the problem
- Common designs for quality improvement
- Before Intervention After design
- Multiple Before Intervention After design
- Factorial experiments with multiple factors
- Enumerative versus analytic studies
- Error proofing/mistake proofing
- Innovation
- What to do after the project is over
- Reporting the results
- Discussion
- Acknowledgment
- References

An article published in 2004 [1] suggests that approximately 7.5% of the 2.5 million hospital admissions in Canada in 2000 resulted in adverse events, 37% of which are preventable; of these, the most responsible service was surgery with 185 (51%) of 360. Clearly, these data suggest that surgery should be the focus of improvement strategies.

Leape [2] suggests that there are many reasons why error has not been properly dealt with in the health care delivery system. Some of the later discussion in this article provides concrete suggestions as to what clinicians, and surgeons in particular, can be doing to make things better for patients and themselves in the health care system.

One hundred thousand lives

As reported by McCue [3], Berwick of the Institute for Health Care Improvement (IHI) made a pledge to save 100,000 lives by 9:00 AM June 14, 2006 by having 1600 hospitals make six changes:

1. Make rapid response teams to prevent patient deterioration.
2. Provide evidence-based care for victims of acute myocardial infarction (AMI) to reduce their mortality.
3. Increase the use of ventilator bundles to prevent ventilator-acquired pneumonia.
4. Increase the use of central line bundles to prevent central line infections.
5. Prevent surgical site infections with preoperative antibiotics.
6. Prevent severe drug events by reconciliation with a list of common drug interactions.

Indeed, more than 3100 hospitals eventually got involved, and there were more than 122,000 lives saved. This provides a glowing example of how hospitals can do simple things to improve the care they provide to patients, their customers.

---

[a] Suite 410, 2000 Credit Valley Road, Mississauga, Ontario L5M 4N4, Canada
[b] Department of Clinical Epidemiology and Biostatistics, McMaster University and Biostatistics Unit, St Joseph's Healthcare Hamilton, Martha H 322, 50 Charlton Avenue East, Hamilton, Ontario L8N 4A6, Canada
* Corresponding author.
E-mail address: goldsmit@mcmaster.ca (C.H. Goldsmith).

Five million lives

Building on the success of the 100,000 lives campaign, Berwick aims to save 5 million lives by December 9, 2008. This is important, because there are 15 million people who are harmed in the US health system annually, or 40,000 per day. This should be accomplished by adding six new ventures to the former six to get the following:

7. Prevent Methicillin-resistant *Staphylococcus aureus* (MRSA) infections.
8. Reduce harm from the high-alert medications: anticoagulants, sedatives, narcotics, and insulin.
9. Reduce surgical complications.
10. Prevent pressure ulcers.
11. Deliver reliable evidence-based care for patients who have congestive heart failure.
12. Get boards on board.

Notice that numbers 3, 4, 5, 7, 8, 9, and 10 could involve surgery and surgeons in various ways.

The IHI has had recent community information calls related to surgery on transforming medical/surgery care (June 18, 2007), on reducing hospital-acquired infections (MRSA/Vancomycin-resistant *Enterococcus* [VRE]/*Clostridium difficile* [*C. diff*]; June 21, 2007), and on reducing surgical complications (June 25, 2007). Each call provided an expert on the telephone call to provide listeners with ideas for quality improvement (QI) at their location and the ability to ask questions about strategy and resources to make the improvement happen. These three calls indicate that attention is being paid to surgery to improve health care for patients. These calls are focused on immediately implementable changes that should result in better care for patients [4].

Safer health care now

In various Canadian provinces, an organization with similar recommendations to the IHI has emerged with six interventions [5]:

1. Create rapid response teams.
2. Improve AMI care.
3. Implement reconciliation of medications.
4. Prevent central line infections.
5. Prevent surgical site infections.
6. Prevent ventilator-associated pneumonia, from their Phase I and have four new interventions.
7. Prevent adverse drug events in long-term care settings.
8. Prevent falls in long-term care.
9. Prevent harm from antibiotic-resistant organisms.
10. Implement appropriate prophylaxis for deep vein thrombosis and pulmonary embolism.

Notice how similar these Canadian recommendations are to those proposed by the IHI.

As an example of what might be improved, the IHI has prepared a starter kit that summarizes what to do to prevent pressure ulcers in your hospital environment [6]. In essence, the IHI recommends six steps:

1. Do a pressure ulcer admission assessment on all patients.
2. Do a daily reassessment of all patients.
3. Inspect all patients' skin daily.
4. Keep all patients dry, and moisturize their skin.
5. Make sure all patients have appropriate nutrition, including hydration.
6. Minimize the pressure on all patients by turning them every 2 hours, and use pressure-relieving surfaces.

The IHI also presents data from benchmarked hospitals that show these ideas do work to reduce pressure ulcers.

How to perform quality improvement clinical research

Traditional clinical research tries to answer original research questions that have not yet been adequately answered with a randomized controlled trial (RCT) to avoid bias. Generally, with QI projects, your team already knows that the solution works in another location; your team must then satisfy itself that it works in your hospital. Another difference is that an RCT can take many years to complete, whereas the typical QI project can often be completed in a few months, and in as few as 100 days in some locations [7]. A strategy for improvement is described next.

FOCUS-PDCA

These acronyms stand for Find a problem to solve or process to improve, Organize a team that knows the process, Clarify current knowledge of the process (if there is a well-researched solution, such as a statistically significant and clinically important method to solve your problem), Understand causes of process variation, and Select the process improvement (FOCUS), and Plan the implementation and continue data collection, Do the improvements, Check the results (sometimes an S for Study), and Act to hold the gains and continue improvement (PDCA). These two acronyms help to keep everyone focused on the problem at hand and keep them paying attention to the steps for continuous QI.

PICOT

PICOT stands for Patients, Intervention, Comparison, Outcome, and Time, which are all components of a good QI question [8] (see the article by Thoma, McKnight, McKay, and Haines in this issue). Each QI project team should state the question that the team is trying to answer with their FOCUS-PDCA cycle. The question should be capable of being spoken in a single breath so that it can serve as a way for all team members to state clearly and simply what they are doing.

For example, in carpal tunnel (CT) surgery, does a strict check sheet to ensure hand washing in 2008 compared with no check sheet in 2007 lower the rate of CT cases with a clinical infection?

What can surgeons do?

Surgeons can develop voluntary error reporting of all errors and even near misses, promote legislation to extend peer review protections to data related to patient safety and QI with no reprisals for error reporting, avoid reliance on memory, avoid reliance on vigilance, and simplify key procedures and standardized work processes. Some progress has been made on mandatory disclosure of errors to patients by clinicians in Manitoba and Quebec in Canada and in various states in the United States [9].

Surgeons should be able to identify areas for safety improvement, adopt computer order entry and computer-assisted decision making, encourage an error-friendly environment for learning from errors, involve learners (medical students, interns, and residents) in studying items for error reduction, make previous actions part of accreditation and funding, form interdisciplinary teams with experts in safety and QI, evaluate all changes with the PDCA cycle, and educate all staff you work with by benchmarking on the best. Finally, surgeons need to "encourage no-fault healing" from errors created by the health care system. There is a need to get the lawyers out of health care and use the medical protective premiums to repair the health care system. A commentary by Levinson and Gallagher [9] mentions that British Columbia has legislation that prevents apologies given by clinicians to patients from being used as an admission of liability, which represents progress toward allaying the fears raised by clinicians who want to participate in improving the system. Surgeons worried about disclosure of errors may be relieved by the suggestions provided in an article on ethics by Hebert and colleagues [10] that suggests error disclosure, apologies, and being told that the problem is going to be fixed lead to fewer lawsuits, because patients expect these acts to be part of the patient/health professional caregiving relationship. Methods of disclosing errors should become part of the training of health professionals [9].

Deming [11], a quality guru, promoted that all work takes place in a system. The system has suppliers and customers, who take what you as workers add to the system. Hence, improvements in the system should involve your suppliers and customers (patients). A second point made by Deming [11] is that there is variation in everything and that a good part of QI is to reduce variation. To do this properly, one needs to understand the system, and this takes knowledge (the complete theory of how the system runs and why) [12,13]. One is always learning about the system by experimentation and adding improvements. Finally, Deming [11] recognized that human psychology was a necessary tool to get workers to improve the system constantly, for their benefit and for that of others. One of Deming's key points about psychology is not to use incentives because they do not work in the long haul [14]; indeed, they usually lead to poorer performance than in their absence.

Once a problem is identified, a team of five to seven key stakeholders should be assembled to tackle the problem. Clearly, at least one should be a surgeon, whereas the others can come from other sectors of the organization that should understand the problem. The other team members should be relevant stakeholders who could also judge the merits of any QI strategy. They might be nurses, physical therapists, internists, supervisors, and patients or their representative. The team should have a QI consultant who is trained at the level of a "Blackbelt" and understands and can teach QI strategies and tools to the team as they are needed [15]. The team and the problem should have the complete support of all senior management of the hospital, particularly the chief executive officer (CEO).

Suppose the proposed solution to the QI problem works somewhere else, also known as benchmarking. The main question for the team is can we make it work here?

Benchmarking the problem

As Camp [16] has eluded, the process of benchmarking has 10 steps that are vague but in essence state that your team should do the following:

1. Identify the process to be improved.
2. Identify other locations where the problem has already been solved.
3. Determine your data collection method and get the data.
4. Determine the gap between how well you do compared with the benchmarked place.
5. Project what level your team would like to make your hospital.
6. Communicate the findings of your benchmark process to the rest of your organization.
7. Establish goals for your QI project.

8. Develop your action plan.
9. Implement your plan and monitor whether it reached the goal.
10. Recalibrate your benchmarks.

In essence, this process suggests that one should look to where the problem has already been solved; try to mimic that performance at your hospital; and if you can in a small way, work to make it happen at all locations in your hospital. Be sure to credit the location that was your benchmark. Note that this does not need to be a traditional RCT. Usually, the method has already been proved, and all there is to show is that it can happen in your hospital culture with the resources and people that you have to work with to get the gain.

As an example, suppose you try to reduce the rate of bed sores in your hospital. This has been put as one of the challenges in the "save 5 million lives" campaign. There should be good-quality evidence, so that all your team needs to do is to see if you can have the same effect in your hospital.

Once your team has tried out the new way of doing things and found out that it does not work, do not implement it as part of the hospital policy. If does work in one location in your hospital, however, try to implement it in the rest of your hospital. Do not be disappointed if the modification does not work; there are many ideas that do not work (trivial many), whereas the few that do work may be quite helpful (vital few) [17].

Common designs for quality improvement

Before Intervention After design

In Fig. 1, the B is the Before measurement of the outcome that indicates quality for your team. Clearly, it is best to make A for After be the same outcome. The I indicates the proposed Intervention should take place long enough to have an impact and between the time when B was collected and when A was collected. Time runs from left to right; thus, T_0 is clearly before T_1. Ideally, the change, A minus B, should be a clinically important improvement; however, although it would be nice to have a statistically significant improvement, this is less important if the effect has been shown in other locations with RCTs and the magnitude of the effect is large enough to be convincing to your team and the management of your hospital to make them want to implement the intervention throughout your hospital. For example, from the PICOT research question, the B could be the rate of infections in 2007, A could be rate of infections in 2008, and I could be the check sheet–verified hand washing implemented between 2007 and 2008.

Multiple Before Intervention After design

In Fig. 2, the two Bs in the title indicate that that there is more than one measure of the outcome done Before the Intervention; ideally, at least k, where k can be as long as the outcome data have been collected since the last process change, possibly in months. Ideally, the multiple measurements should be shown to be in control with a control chart [18] to be used as a stable estimate of the outcome before implementing the Intervention. Although the After measurement could be repeated multiple times after the Intervention, this is usually the case if the final step of the PDCA cycle is properly implemented. The final step A here is the Act step, which means the hospital should be measuring the outcome regularly to make sure that it does not drift back to the Before level and that the culture of the hospital knows that there is a new way of doing things. The statistical analysis here is to compare the A outcomes with the B outcomes to determine if there is a credible and clinically relevant improvement. It is hoped that After minus Before could also be shown to be statistically significant. The results should be shared with everyone in the hospital. For example, from the PICOT research question, there could be many years from which the annual infection rates would be computed, say 2000 to 2007; the Intervention could still

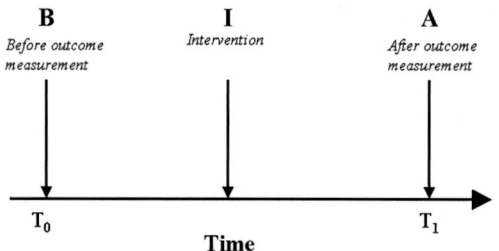

Fig. 1. Before intervention after (BIA) design. T_0 represents the time of the before outcome measurement. T_1 represents the time of the after outcome measurement.

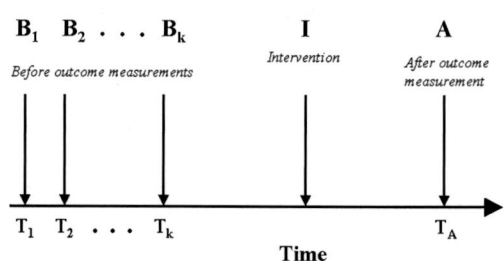

Fig. 2. Multiple before intervention after (BBIA) design. T_1, T_2, ...T_k represent the times of the before outcome measurements B_1, B_2, ...B_k. T_A represents the time of the after outcome measurement.

be the check sheet hand-washing policy implemented between 2007 and 2008, whereas the After measures could be the years 2008 and annually thereafter to see that the reduced annual infection rates were maintained.

Factorial experiments with multiple factors

Factorial designs seem to be little used in health care; however, they are particularly useful when there are many factors that could have an impact on the quality measure of the process being improved. The Blackbelt consultant should understand how to use such designs and help to advise how to plan, conduct, and analyze such designs to determine the important few factors [17] from the trivial many that could be involved. Most factorial designs should be conducted as RCTs [19]. For example, suppose there were two factors to be implemented in the CT operations (Fig. 3). One factor could be check sheet hand washing or not, whereas the second factor could be preoperative antibiotics or not. The factorial design would have four groups: (1) check sheet hand washing, antibiotics; (2) check sheet hand washing, no antibiotics; (3) no check sheet hand washing, antibiotics; and (4) no check sheet hand washing, no antibiotics. These four groups should be randomly assigned to eligible patients who undergo CT surgery with a balanced allocation; the infection rates in subsequent months could then be used to evaluate which of the two factors or their interaction was needed to lower the infection rates. The outcome measurements, OM_1 and OM_2, represent that the intervention effects might be measured more than once or that more than one outcome might be measured at the same time.

An editorial by Perneger [20] in 2006 suggests that it still might be better if more QI studies were done as RCTs. The authors agree, but the team doing the study has to decide whether it is worthwhile to do an RCT. Perneger [20] suggests 10 reasons that make an RCT preferable to doing some form of before/after study; however, the time to conceive, carry out, and analyze the RCT may be much longer than other before/after designs.

Enumerative versus analytic studies

Traditional statistical principles are taught using enumerative methods, wherein probability and sampling of closed frames have their genesis. Conversely, a process cannot have its future sampled; as such, it is called an analytic study. Such processes need to be in control before the principles of enumerative statistics can be applied to them. Checking to see if the process is in control has been solved using control charts. There are as many as eight patterns that are unlikely to happen when the process is in control. If some unusual patterns are detected, they are labeled as special causes and removed from the system, leaving what would be an in-control process, with common cause variation. This in-control process can then be used for prediction of the future. Experiments on the process can be used to reduce the common cause variation so that fewer patients get into trouble because of unusual events that may cause error.

For example, the weekly infection rate data could be put through a P control chart to see if the infection rates in the hospital at which the QI project is to be done are in control. If they are in control, implementing the QI hand-washing project can use these data as a baseline in the before intervention after (BIA) design if warranted.

Error proofing/mistake proofing

Grout [21] lists more than 150 ways that a health care system can be made more mistake-proof. Many of these ideas have already been used in health care and surgery; however, not every hospital has these strategies in place. Indeed, if an error happens, there are some general principles that should be considered to correct these errors in the future. Move knowledge out of people's heads into the world to prevent the error from happening again. Detect and correct the mistake before it has an impact on a patient, possibly by stopping the process that led to the error and reducing the effect of the error. People have trouble with tasks that have lots of alternative choices; thus, reducing the

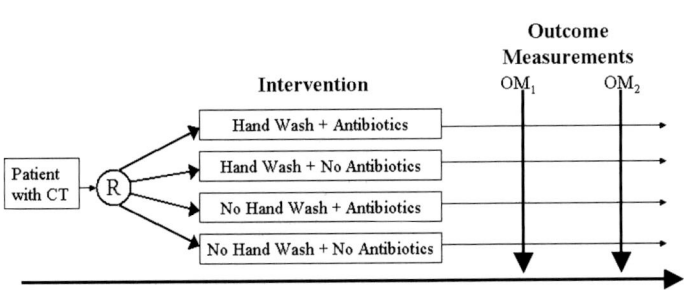

Fig. 3. Factorial experiments with multiple factors (FEMFs). OM_1 indicates outcome measurement 1; OM_2, outcome measurement 2; R, randomization.

choices and number of alternatives for each choice often prevents errors. Simplifying the system leads to fewer errors. The system should be visible to make sure that the right thing does happen when it should, on time, and each time throughout all shifts of personnel. If an error cannot be anticipated, mistake-proofing does not lead to stopping it from happening. If one claims an improvement, the evidence may exist that the past was error-prone and make some hospitals and people fear being sued for what they did in the past. Here is another place wherein we do not want the lawyers to be involved because this does not provide for the opportunities to improve the process. If the process is not in control, it is going to be difficult to mistake-proof it. The process must be predictable. We should convert a blame-oriented culture into one that is a just and fair culture. Surgeons should indelibly sign the site of surgery before the patient is draped to make sure that the proper site is cut open. MRI scans could all have metal detectors to pick up those metal pieces that patients have forgotten to mention. Patients should be told in each hospital that it is acceptable to ask all health professionals if they have washed their hands before examining the patient.

Innovation

Innovation [22] is taking an idea from one location and making it work with the resources and people in another site. Inventive problem-solving methods [22] access all of the theory of mathematics, physics, chemistry, and other sciences and try to present them as possible solutions associated with 41 principles of problem solving. One such principle is to make things that are symmetric into an asymmetry to see if that strategy improves an outcome. A second such principle is to change the order of tasks in a procedure to determine if the changed order leads to improvement. These should be consulted for innovative solutions to problems that the properly structured stakeholder team could evaluate with a FOCUS-PDCA cycle to see if it leads to a better solution.

Cook and colleagues [23] show how a five-step process can lead to change of a clinician's behavior. The steps include (1) an environmental scan, (2) understand the current behavior, (3) target the behavior for change, (4) adopt effective behavioral change methods, and (5) synergize the process of change. It is interesting that their language is devoid of many QI terms; however, the direction of the intent is much like that of the FOCUS-PDCA cycle. Almost an entire issue of the *Journal of Critical Care* [2005;34(4)] [24] is taken up with how this strategy was used to change the use of thromboprophylaxis in a network of Canadian intensive care units (ICUs) from around 60% to greater than 90% of the appropriate patients. Although such a high rate is not unknown in patients who have had major orthopedic surgery [25], the improvement shows what can be done without using an RCT but putting to bear appropriate QI methods.

What to do after the project is over

Once you complete your QI project, you want to take advantage of the fact that you helped it to happen. You should have been an advocate for making it happen.

If it has worked at your hospital, be an advocate for making it happen elsewhere. This can be done by listing it on your department or personal Web site, writing about it in your department newsletter, and writing about it for *Quality Progress* (QP). QP is looking for health care articles that show how QI principles have led to improvements in quality. Present it at a surgical meeting locally, nationally, and internationally.

Reporting the results

This article has shown that QI can play a role in improving the health care that our patients deserve. Surgeons can show some of their leadership skills in helping to solve the QI problems that are badly in need of solution in our health care system.

Discussion

Surgeons are recognized leaders in the health professional hierarchy, and as such, they should be the ones to step forward and lead the health QI charge to care for patients better. Surgeons need to work on teams in their local environments to help make things better by using fewer resources and, at the same time, making health care better for all involved, especially the patients. Although the path to improvement is not going to occur overnight, the journey should be satisfying for those who participate in that they tried to make the system better than it was before they were added to it. This is the mark of a true professional.

Acknowledgment

The authors thank Leslie McKnight for helping with the graphs shown in this article.

References

[1] Baker GR, Norton PG, Flintoft V, et al. The Canadian Adverse Events Study: the incidence of

adverse events among hospital patients in Canada. CMAJ 2004;170(11):1678–86.
[2] Leape LL. Error in medicine. JAMA 1994;272(23): 1851–7. Response letters. JAMA 1995;274(6): 457–61.
[3] McCue M. Commentary: Converting political fervor for the benefit of everyone. If everyone were half as adamant about improving healthcare as they were about partisan politics, we'd all be safer. And "I'm losing my patience": Donald Berwick. Managed Healthcare Executive. February 2005. Available at: www.managedhealthcareexecutive.com. Accessed November 19, 2007.
[4] Available at: www.ihi.org/IHI/Programs/IMPACT Network/IMPACTNetwork.htm? Accessed August 8, 2007.
[5] Available at: www.saferhealthcarenow.ca. Accessed August 8, 2007.
[6] Available at: www.ihi.org/IHI/Programs/Campaign. Accessed April 1, 2007.
[7] Barry R, Smith AC. The Manager's guide to six sigma in healthcare. Practical tips and tools for improvement. Milwaukee (WI): ASQ Quality Press; 2005.
[8] Haynes RB, Sackett DL, Guyatt GH, et al. Clinical epidemiology. How to do clinical practice research. 3rd edition. New York: Lippincott Williams & Wilkins; 2006.
[9] Levinson W, Gallagher TH. Disclosing medical errors to patients: a status report in 2007. CMAJ 2007;177(3):265–7.
[10] Hebert PC, Levin AV, Robertson G. Bioethics for clinicians 23: disclosure of medical error. CMAJ 2001;164(4):509–13.
[11] Deming WE. Out of the crisis. Center for Advanced Engineering Study. Cambridge (MA): MIT Press; 1986. Cambridge University Press; 1988.
[12] Senge PM. The fifth discipline. The art and practice of the learning organization. New York: Doubleday/Currency; 1990.
[13] Senge PM, Kleiner A, Roberts C, et al. The fifth discipline fieldbook. Strategies and tools for building a learning organization. New York: Doubleday/Currency; 1994.
[14] Kohn A. Punished by rewards. The trouble with gold stars, incentive plans, A's, praise and other bribes. Boston: Houghton Mifflin Company; 1999.
[15] Pyzdek T. The six stigma handbook. A complete guide for Greenbelts, Blackbelts, & Managers at all levels. New York: McGraw-Hill; 2001.
[16] Camp RC. Benchmarking. The search for industry best practices that lead to superior performance. Milwaukee (WI): ASQC Quality Press; 1989.
[17] Juran JM. The non-Pareto principle; mea culpa. Qual Prog 1975;8(5):8–9.
[18] Brassard M, Field C, Oddo F, et al. The problem solving memory jogger. Seven steps to improved processes. Salem (NH): GOAL/QPC; 2000.
[19] Montgomery DC. Design and analysis of experiments. 5th edition. Toronto: J Wiley & Sons Inc; 2001.
[20] Perneger T. Ten reasons to conduct a randomized study in quality improvement. Int J Qual Health Care 2006;18(6):395–6.
[21] Grout J. Mistake-proofing the design of healthcare processes. AHRQ publication no. 07-0020. Rockville (MD): Agency for Healthcare Research and Quality; May 2007. Available at: www.ahrq.gov. If you have a new idea for mistake proofing, then it can be submitted to www.mistakeproofing.com/medical. Accessed November 19, 2007.
[22] Altshuller GS. (Altov H), translated by Shulyak L. And suddenly the inventor appeared. TRIZ, the theory of inventive problem solving. 2nd edition. Worcester (MA): Technical Innovation Center, Inc; 1996.
[23] Cook DJ, Montori VM, McMullin JP, et al. Improving patients' safety locally: challenging clinician behaviour. Lancet 2004;363:1224–30.
[24] Issue of the Journal of Critical Care 2005;34(4).
[25] Campbell SE, Walker AE, Grimshaw JM, et al. The prevalence of prophylaxis for deep vein thrombosis in acute hospital trusts. Int J Qual Health Care 2001;13(4):309–16.

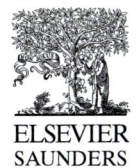

How to Become a Successful Clinical Investigator

Achilleas Thoma, MD, MSc, FRCS(C), FACS[a,b,c,*], Ted Haines, MD, MSc, FRCPC[a], Eric Duku, MSc, PStat[d], Leslie McKnight, MSc[b], Charlie Goldsmith, BSc, MSc, PhD[a,c,e]

- Preconditions for academic success
  Mentoring
  The role of the periodic priority list
  Time management (protected time)
- Methodologic training
- Moving from a "mentee" role to independent investigator (going out on one's own)
- Is it possible to fit in both family and an academic career?
- Summary
- References

The purpose of this article is to help residents, fellows, and junior faculty who aspire for an academic career, and seasoned plastic surgeons who may wish to have a second "lease on life," to become successful clinical investigators. It is of particular relevance to those who love the intellectual challenge of research, and are keen to find answers to clinically important problems in plastic surgery.

Successful clinical investigators are the primary investigators of important clinical research, the lead authors of high impact publications, recipients of career awards and honors in their profession, and eventually leaders in their field. It is never too late to become a successful clinical investigator: all it takes is passion and initiative.

There are tangible benefits to being a clinical investigator. In conjunction with the high quality clinical care you provide your patients is the opportunity to educate medical students, residents, and colleagues. In addition, there is the prospect of working in a stimulating environment with young minds, finding answers to clinically important questions, or dismantling entrenched dogmas passed on by the so called "experts" of a previous generation of plastic surgeons.

---

[a] Department of Clinical Epidemiology and Biostatistics, McMaster University, Hamilton Health Sciences Centre, 1200 Main Street West, Hamilton, ON L8N 3Z5, Canada
[b] Department of Surgery, Division of Plastic Surgery, McMaster University, St. Joseph's Healthcare, 50 Charlton Avenue East, Hamilton, ON L8N 4A6, Canada
[c] Surgical Outcomes Research Centre (SOURCE), McMaster University, St. Joseph's Healthcare, 50 Charlton Avenue East, Hamilton, ON L8N 4A6, Canada
[d] Department of Psychiatry and Behavioural Neurosciences, Offord Centre for Child Studies, McMaster University, Chedoke Division, Patterson Building Room 217, 1200 Main Street West, Hamilton, ON L8N 3Z5, Canada
[e] Biostatistics Unit, 3rd Floor Martha, Room H322, St. Joseph's Healthcare Hamilton, 50 Charlton Avenue East, Hamilton, ON L8N 4A6, Canada
* Corresponding author. 206 James Street South, Suite 101, Hamilton, ON L8P 3A9, Canada
E-mail address: athoma@mcmaster.ca (A. Thoma).

Preconditions for academic success

The motivations for a clinician to become a clinical investigator will vary, depending on their circumstances, specialty, and interests. Plastic surgeons may not be happy with a routine and unchallenging clinical practice and may wish to pursue the challenge of scholarship.

Various factors have been identified that prevent clinicians from becoming clinical investigators, such as competing clinical service demands, lack of methodologic training necessary to conduct clinical research, lack of mentorship, and other unique factors relevant to their own specific specialty [1–4]. In 1994, the Institute of Medicine identified five main obstacles to careers in clinical research: a lack of protected time, insufficient formal methodologic training, lack of mentors, student debt, and academic emphasis on cellular or molecular research over patient-oriented research [5]. In a later publication, Sackett [6,7] narrowed this list and espoused that academic success as a clinician-scientist is predicated on three preconditions: mentoring, the periodic priority list, and time management. These preconditions for academic success will be discussed in detail.

Mentoring

Mentorship can be defined as "a dynamic, reciprocal relationship in a work environment between an advanced career incumbent (mentor) and a beginner (mentee/protégé), aimed at promoting the development of both" [8]. Mentorship is a common theme in publications addressing the present topic, and is considered essential to one's success. For example, graduates in internal medicine research fellowships were five times more likely to publish at least one paper, and were three times more likely to be principal investigators on a funded research grant, if they had an influential mentor during their fellowship [9]. We can speculate that this "mentor factor" also applies to plastic surgery. In addition, in a survey of faculty from 24 United States medical schools, faculty members with mentors had significantly higher career-satisfaction scores than those without mentors (mean score, 62.6 versus 59.5 on a scale that varies from a low of 20 to a high of 100; $P < 0.003$) [10], and having a mentor was associated with a higher likelihood of promotion to professor [11].

Despite the known benefits of mentoring, few junior faculty members feel as though they have a true mentor. A study that surveyed junior faculty at the University of Washington found that 36% felt that they had mentors [12]. In a more recent systematic review, less than 20% of faculty members had a mentor. Additionally, women perceived that they had more difficulty finding mentors than their male colleagues [13].

It is unclear from the various published reports why the mentoring system is not working well in academic centers. The authors can only speculate that the leadership in many institutions has not recognized the critical role of the mentor and embedded it in the vision plans of the center (or program). Other possibilities could be: the obstinacy of the young faculty member to admit that he or she needs a mentor, thinking they can do it alone; or, the competitive atmosphere in which the young faculty member is working in may make the mentor-protégé relationship not possible.

Finding the right mentor

Finding the right mentor is crucial. "Mentors need to be congenial persons who have had a variety of successful teaching experiences, who have also had success in research, grantsmanship and publication, and who have demonstrated common sense, discretion and good judgment in their service to the institution and in their relationships with graduate students, colleagues and administrators" [14]. The important considerations when selecting a mentor are found in Box 1.

The ideal mentor will provide resources, opportunities, advice, and protection (Table 1). The mentor should provide you with the resources you will need early on in your career, such as space to work, free photocopying, secretarial or research

---

Box 1: Important considerations when selecting a mentor

1. The mentor should be a competent plastic surgeon clinical investigator who understands your career at your institution, university, or hospital.
2. The mentor must have achieved his or her own academic success and must be comfortable taking a back seat to those being mentored in matters of authorship, and not compete with you for recognition.
3. The mentor should not directly control your academic appointment or your base salaries.
4. The mentor must be willing to devote the time and energy to assist you in both routine and unexpected academic and personal challenges
5. You must provide periodic feedback to your mentor to ensure he or she remains the best person capable to continue mentoring you.

Data from Sackett DL. On the determinants of academic success as a clinician-scientist. Clin Invest Med 2001;24:94–100; and Haynes RB, Sackett DL, Guyatt GH, et al. Clinical Epidemiology 3rd Edition. Philadelphia: Lippincott Williams & Wilkins; 2006.

Table 1: **The ideal roles of a mentor**

	Key roles
Resources	Office space and supplies (eg, photocopying, internet access) Secretarial and administrative support Financial support to attend meetings, conferences, courses Research coordinator support

Opportunities	Assisting the mentors with:
	  Ongoing research projects for "hands on" experience and writing manuscripts for publication,
	  Reviewing manuscripts and grant applications
	  Comparing notes to sharpen appraisal skills,
	  Attending meetings and making "connections"
	  Learning how ethics review committees, and grant review committees work
	  Joining scientific committees (ie, grant review committees, task forces to writing guidelines)

Advice	Unhurried safe opportunities to think through academic and social development and to discuss methodologic challenges of projects, pros and cons of working with particular collaborators, balancing professional and social life
Protection	Practicing presentations and defending your conclusions in a friendly atmosphere, before presenting at a national meeting. Guarding against criticism from other investigators who may be protecting "turf"

Data from Sackett DL. On the determinants of academic success as a clinician-scientist. Clin Invest Med 2001;24:94–100; and Haynes RB, Sackett DL, Guyatt GH, et al. Clinical Epidemiology 3rd Edition. Philadelphia: Lippincott Williams & Wilkins; 2006.

coordinator support, and the opportunity to collaborate on research projects. The mentor should provide you with the opportunities to review grants and manuscripts sent to him or her for consideration, which will help you sharpen your critical appraisal skills [6,7]. Your mentor should introduce you to the functions of the Institutional Research Review Boards, grant review committees, and let you coauthor articles for publication. He or she will support your attendance at scientific meetings and introduce you to other clinical investigators with whom you may interact in the future.

The mentor should not off-load on you their undesired tasks, but instead bring you on board with the on-going research projects, so you can gain a hands-on experience and learn to function in a collaborative team. Although it would be ideal to interact face-to-face with mentors and collaborators, the availability of the internet and electronic communication make it such that collaboration with mentors from other cities and countries is possible if local expertise is lacking.

All in all, the authors believe that mentoring is an important precondition to being a successful investigator and the available evidence seems to support this. For Divisions or Departments of Plastic Surgery, mentoring is crucial. There is evidence in other areas of medicine to suggest that the retention of young faculty in an academic organization is positively correlated with the formation of preceptor partnerships. One study showed that 38% of junior faculty who did not form such preceptor partnership left the organization, compared with with 15% of those who formed one [15]. A more recent systematic review on mentoring in academic medicine identified an apparent effect of mentoring on research career guidance, productivity, and success [13].

The role of the periodic priority list

Sackett [6] suggested that the person being mentored should present to his or her mentor a periodic priority list. This priority list remains central to the academic success throughout the rest of one's career. This priority list has four parts or sublists:

Part 1 includes those things that you are doing and should quit. It also includes those things you have been asked to do and don't want to do.
Part 2 includes those things you are not doing and want to start.
Part 3 includes the things you want to keep doing.
Part 4 addresses how to plan to shorten the list in part 1 and lengthen list in part 2.

You can generate lists by reviewing your diary intermittently and pruning items (activities) listed in part 1. The part 2 list should be the exciting one.

Ideas come from various sources, such as the next research question that follows the answer to your last one, and ideas generated from patient problems or discussion with colleagues or after attending a meeting or research gatherings. The purpose of the periodic priority lists is to prevent burnout and to make it fun to go to work.

The major roles of a university faculty member are education, research, service and administration. While most plastic surgeons are overwhelmed by the service part of their jobs, the other three areas deserve some consideration in career planning and, hence, discussion with your mentor. What do you want to do as an educator? Do you want to train residents in plastic surgery? Convince medical students to pursue a career in surgery, particularly plastics? Have graduate students, such as MSc and PhD students, help pursue in depth topics that are of interest to you, or have residents do portions of research topics of interest to you? Many of these tasks will require you to supervise these learners and that will need some planning and time; putting further pressure on your scarce resource of time. The research part of your life should be the major focus of your time with your mentor. This area is the most difficult part to get under proper control, so it does not swamp the rest of your life. Every faculty member is expected to do some administration. Of which committees in your hospital, university, and professional societies do you see yourself as a member? These may need to be planned in your life. A 5-year plan for your education, research, and administration would be a worthwhile discussion with your mentor. This should be visited annually with your mentor, to keep them up to date with new opportunities.

Time management (protected time)

The most important element of time management for academic success is setting aside and ruthlessly protecting time that is spent writing for publication [6]. A good author to read as a new faculty member is Boice [16], who has counseled many faculty members over the years, and helped them get their life organized to be successful as a faculty member. The key message of his book is to keep everything, including your writing, in moderation. Most surgeons presume that this protected time occurs outside normal working hours, such as weekends, holidays, or late evenings after busy clinical regular hours. However, this type of activity takes its toll on the investigator's family and friends. Furthermore, if you are exhausted from seeing a large number of patients in busy clinics, it is highly unlikely you will have any physical stamina, let alone creativity to work on a manuscript late in the evening. Successful academic surgeons set aside 1 day per week for research activities. During this time, they are not burdened by clinical responsibilities or other interruptions. It is imperative that no interruptions occur on your writing days.

The ideal environment for writing will be one where there are as few interruptions as possible. Box 2 shows the activities that can subvert the protected time for clinical research.

Lack of protected time is detrimental for clinical investigators. One study found that each increase in 10 hours of clinical work a week was associated with a 23% decrease in the odds of having federal or nonprofit grant support [17].

In plastic surgery, finding time is possible only if surgeons work in a group setting, with colleagues who have similar interests and are willing to cover for each other's patients while those surgeons are working on a clinical research project or a manuscript. There is nothing more detrimental to clinical research than an interruption to deal with a complication of one of your patients. This type of interruption consumes time, such as waiting for a patient to arrive and eventually see in a crowded emergency room; waiting for lab results, or x-rays; or waiting for other specialists to assist your patient and make a decision on care. If you work in a collaborative group practice, your patient becomes your colleagues' patient and they will assume the emergency care if necessary. If your work is subspecialized, such as perforator flap breast reconstruction or head and neck reconstruction, then you should identify colleagues with the same skills who are familiar with your practice and patients and support each other. They can address any conceivable problem that can arise. This may be simplified further if these same colleagues were assisting you in these cases and are familiar with any technical nuances

---

Box 2: Advice for protecting research time

1. Do not carry your pager.
2. Do not check your e-mail.
3. Do not let your friends, colleagues, residents, or fellows know where you are.
4. Do not allow your secretary to divulge your whereabouts, except for a critical emergency that cannot be handled by one of your colleagues, or in the case of a family emergency.
5. Do not review manuscripts during your protected time.
6. Do not use your research time to catch up on journals.
7. Do not work in an environment where the phone rings all the time (preferably unplug it, but ensure your secretary can find you in a true emergency).

or problems that may have arisen in the initial surgery.

What if there are no other plastic surgeons in your academic department or hospital? This scenario is less likely, but if it occurs you will need to make an arrangement with other surgeons from the community to cover your cases while you write. Another model, as suggested by Boice [16] (his Nihil Numus idea) is to learn to write in small amounts without setting aside days at a time. Everyone has gaps in their lives, such as 10-minute periods that can be used for writing. The accumulations of multiple, daily 10-minute periods over, for example, a week, can add up to more than you might accomplish in a single writing day.

Competition in practice is a detriment to research productivity. Invariably, if an income differential enters into the equation, it will destroy collaboration. A plastic surgeon, whose only interest is to see more and more patients and augment his income, will not wish to share his revenues with a colleague who locks himself or herself in a room to write yet another manuscript. It is important therefore, that each plastic surgeon in the collaborative group sets one working day aside, which will be respected by all the members of the group.

If some members of an academic group are not interested in clinical research and prefer to see patients only, then the Division Chief should make it absolutely clear what the remunerative compensation formula will be. This formula should be explicit, and all members of the division should "buy into it" to avoid a later misunderstanding. The formula needs to take into account some credit for writing and the other academic tasks, not just clinical work.

The amount of protected time that a successful clinical investigator should aim for is not clearly delineated. Elta [1] suggests that protected time should be 50% in academic gastroenterology. It is highly unlikely for a Division or Department of Plastic Surgery to be able to take much time out of the pressure cooker of clinical demands, when this specialty is already experiencing such a shortage of trained personnel, especially in emergency coverage [18]. Plastic surgeons who may be interested in devoting more than just a day a week to clinical research should apply for provincial or state or federal career awards to support their research activities. In some institutions they may have the opportunity to be recipients of a "Chair" in a particular line of work.

Methodologic training

Feeling ignorant about methodologic techniques and statistics make surgeons hesitant to work collaboratively with investigators. To facilitate clinical research productivity it is imperative to acquire some skills in health research methodology. For those who have no such training, they should work collaboratively in a team setting where such expertise exists. In other words, there should be pairing of clinicians and investigators to compliment the expertise of each member.

For new faculty clinical researchers, the authors recommend obtaining formal research training on study design, statistical analysis, and database and outcome study techniques. Various methods of acquiring methodologic training are given in Box 3.

Moving from a "mentee" role to independent investigator (going out on one's own)

The transition from the position of junior faculty clinical investigator to independent investigator requires some thoughtful planning. The junior faculty member needs to learn the local promotion rules. The promotion rules from an assistant to full professor level vary considerably among academic centers. It is imperative early on to start and maintain a clinical, educational, and research dossier that carefully lists your contribution to your division or program. Discuss the creation of these documents with your mentor. Each university has its own guidelines to be followed and often you will have many questions as to format and content.

It is important to establish your own research ideas early in the new job and commence exploring them as soon as possible. Any delay or procrastination in this endeavor will lead you down the unwanted path of a busy clinical practice, with overbooked clinics that can be unrelenting and all consuming.

In addition to working with a mentor, you should also consider developing networks with

---

Box 3: Various approaches to acquiring research methodologic training

- MSc or PhD programs in the areas of Health Research Methodology, Health Sciences, Clinical Epidemiology, and Biostatistics
- Academic research groups, such as Surgical Outcomes Research Center (SOURCE) at McMaster University, Hamilton, Ontario Canada
- Industry sponsored or institutional seminars, workshops, and training courses
- National and international peer-reviewed scientific meetings
- Grant preparation workshops
- Undergraduate or graduate courses in statistics, computing, and software

other colleagues from your own specialty or other specialties with whom you can collaborate. You should also familiarize yourself with the local resources that may be available to you in your institution. Find out if your Department of Surgery provides clinical research support programs, such as full or part-time study coordinators who can help you with long or short-term projects. Most importantly, find out as much information as possible about the central liaison office for granting agencies, which can provide you with the information on the appropriate grant agencies to which you may be applying for your next project. Your academic department may provide small research grants, which can be used for pilot projects. With some early findings, you can then apply to a larger competitive external source.

With the progression to an independent research grant, you will have proven that you have moved to the independent investigator status. An important message here, however, is that even if you have reached this milestone in your career, you should never work in isolation. Work in teams and tap the expertise of your colleagues. Meaningful work is rarely produced by individual effort!

You should take the opportunity to present your research ideas to your peers at local, national, and international meetings. Try to concentrate on those meetings that use a peer review process. After you get some experience with the meetings, try to organize sessions on topics of interest to you, where you organize the session as well as present your work. This is a way to become visible in the academic community. It also helps with your writing, if you have to prepare a draft paper for the meeting and can benefit from the comments of your peers on your research. As you progress in your career, try to present only at those meetings where you have been invited or are the keynote speaker. The real currency is published manuscripts in the peer-reviewed literature, not presenting at meetings, although the latter can help move along your publications. Make sure you write as a paper as many of the talks that you give, and submit them for publication to an appropriate peer-reviewed journal. Decide how many invited presentations you think would be enough in a year to not detract you from your main tasks of writing; your mentor could help with this.

Is it possible to fit in both family and an academic career?

In a study of medical school faculty, significant differences in career advancement were identified between women with children and men with children [19]. The time periods in life for having children and career advancement coincide. This inevitably involves compromises both at work and at home. Although quality time with children is important, quantity also counts. In general, women confront this dilemma, whereas men do not; hence, many working mothers feel guilt [1]. This sobering study implies that women who choose to combine an academic medical career with having a family may see their career suffer. Some suggestions offered for women who consider an academic career are the following:

> Choose a partner carefully: one who is willing to share family responsibilities.
> Try to live close to work. Jugglers need to keep their balls close.
> Be sure to hire help for noncritical household chores [1].

As gender inequalities exist in raising children, given the special challenges that women face in academic careers, mentors need to be prepared to assist and advise in this area [20].

Although only 20% of female academics in one study stated it was important to have a mentor of the same gender [21], it is important that female plastic surgeons who wish to become clinical investigators have easy access to female plastic surgeons who can act as additional mentors, and can receive input and advice on issues, such as pregnancy timing, parental leave, part-time appointment, sharing practices, and delegation of household duties.

Because female physicians may be most productive between the ages of 50 and 60 years, they do not fit the career trajectory assumed in promotion policies. It is important therefore, to rethink the issue of promotion in female clinical investigators. This requires active faculty development and visionary policy change, for example, by using a tenure rollback "Stop-the-Clock" option [22,23]. If your university does not have such a policy, try to convince your department to support one. If this meets resistance, then the female academics should organize one with the help of their male colleagues.

Summary

The main preconditions for academic success include:

1. Mentoring
2. Periodic priority lists
3. Time management
4. Methodological training
5. Balancing family life and work

References

[1] Elta GH. How to succeed in academic gastroenterology. Gastrointest Endosc 2006;64:29–30.

[2] Mukamal KJ, Smetana GW, Delbanco T. Clinicians, educators, and investigators in general internal medicine: bridging the gaps. J Gen Intern Med 2002;17:565-71.

[3] Ringel SP, Steiner JF, Vickrey BG, et al. Training clinical researchers in neurology: we must do better. Neurology 2001;57:388-92.

[4] Rossini AA, Greiner DL. Diabetes research in jeopardy: the extinction of clinical diabetes researchers. Ann NY Acad Sci 2007;1103:33-44.

[5] Kelly WN. Careers in clinical research. In: Randolph MA, editor. Obstacles and opportunities. Washington DC: National Academy Press; 1994.

[6] Sackett DL. On the determinants of academic success as a clinician-scientist. Clin Invest Med 2001;24:94-100.

[7] Haynes RB, Sackett DL, Guyatt GH, et al. Clinical Epidemiology. 3rd edition. Philadelphia: Lippincott Williams & Wilkins; 2006.

[8] Healy CC, Welchert AJ. Mentoring relations: a definition to advance research and education. Educ Res 1990;19:17-21.

[9] Steiner JF, Lanphear BP, Curtis P, et al. Indicators of early research productivity among primary care fellows. J Gen Intern Med 2002;17:845-51.

[10] Palepu A, Friedman RH, Barnett RC, et al. Junior faculty members' mentoring relationships and their professional development in U.S. medical schools. Acad Med 1998;73(3):318-23.

[11] Wise MR, Shapiro H, Bodley J, et al. Factors affecting academic promotion in obstetrics and gynecology in Canada. J Obstet Gynaecol Can 2004;26:127-36.

[12] Chew LD, Watanabe JM, Buchwald D, et al. Junior faculty's perspectives on mentoring. Acad Med 2003;78:652.

[13] Sambunjak D, Stauss SE, Marusic A. Mentoring in academic medicine: a systematic review. JAMA 2006;296:1103-15.

[14] XXX Canadian Federation for the Humanities and Social Sciences. The academy as community: a manual of best practices for meeting the needs of new scholars. Ottawa: Canadian Federation for the Humanities and Social Sciences; 2004.

[15] Benson CA, Morahan PS, Sachdeva AK, et al. Effective faculty preceptoring and mentoring during reorganization of an academic medical center. Med Teach 2002;24:550-7.

[16] Boice R. Advice for New Faculty Members. Nihil Nimus. Toronto: Allyn and Bacon; 2000.

[17] Lee TH, Ognibene FP, Schwartz JS. Correlates of external research support among respondents to the 1990 American federation for clinical research survey. Clin Res 1991;39:135-44.

[18] Macadam SA, Kennedy S, Lalonde D, et al. The Canadian plastic surgery workforce survey: interpretation and implications. Plast Reconstr Surg 2007;119(7):2299-306.

[19] Carr PL, Ash AS, Friedman RH, et al. Relation of family responsibilities and gender to the productivity and career satisfaction of medical faculty. Ann Intern Med 1998;129:532-8.

[20] Mason MA, Goulden M. Do babies matter: the effect of family formation on the life long careers of women. Academe 2002;88:21-7.

[21] Levinson W, Kaufman K, Clark B, et al. Mentors and role models for women in academic medicine. West J Med 1991;154:423-6.

[22] Fox G, Schwartz A, Hart K. Work-family balance and academic advancement in medical schools. Acad Psychiatry 2006;30:227-34.

[23] American Council on Education. An agenda for excellence: creating flexibility in tenure-track faculty careers. Sloan foundation, 2005. The executive summary is Available at: http://www.acenet.edu/bookstore/pdf/2005_tenure_flex_summary.pdf. Accessed September 12, 2007.

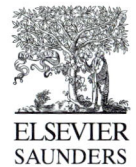

Index

Note: Page numbers of article titles are in **boldface** type.

A

Aesthetic surgery, clinical research in, **269–284**
    measurement of outcomes in, 270–271
    outcome instruments and, 272
    recent outcomes studies in, 271–273
    study design in, 270
Agency for Healthcare Research and Quality categories of outcomes studies, 248
American Society of Anaesthesiologists (ASA) score, 232
Australian/Canadian Osteoarthritis Hand Index, 245

B

Breast surgery, clinical research in, case studies in, 216
    clinical relevancy of, evaluation of, 222–223
    cohort studies in, 216
    efficacy, effectiveness, and efficiency in, 223
    evidence-based surgery approach in, 222–223
    levels of evidence in, 223
    measurement of, new directions in, 222
        outcomes of, 218–219
        rigorous, 221–222
    patient-reported outcome measures in, 219–221
    randomized clinical trials in, 218
    reduction and postmastectomy reconstruction, **215–226**
    study designs in previous studies and, 216–218
    terms used in, 217
Burn Association/Shriners Hospitals for Children Burn Outcomes Questionnaire, 0–5 years form, 11–18 adolescent form, and 15–18 years form, 258
Burns, children with, questionnaire to measure quality of life issues in, 257

C

Carpal Tunnel Questionnaire, 245
Case-controlled studies, and cohort studies, in surgical decision making, 198–200
Child health and illness profile, 255
Child health questionnaire, 255
Child Oral Health Quality of Life Questionnaire,
    Child Perceptions Questionnaire, 8–10 years, 260
        Child Perceptions Questionnaire, 11–14 years, 260
        Child Perceptions Questionnaire Short Forms, 11–14 years, 260
        Parent-Child Perceptions Questionnaire, 6–14 years, 260
Children, treated by plastic surgeons, quality-of-life instruments, with condition-specific measures in, 258–261
Clinical investigator, benefits of, 305
    family issues and, 310
    going out on own, 309–310
    mentoring of, 306
    methodologic training for, 309
    periodic priority list of, 307–308
    roles of mentor, 307
    selection of mentor, 306–307
    successful, how to become, **305–311**
        preconditions for, 306
    time management and, 308–309
Clinical research, in breast surgery, reduction and postmastectomy reconstruction. See *Breast surgery, clinical research in.*
    in head and neck reconstruction. See *Head and neck, reconstruction of, clinical reasearch in.*
Clinical research and practice, narrative reviews in, 208
    systemic reviews in, role of, **207–214**
    types of, 208–209
Cohort studies, and case-controlled studies, in surgical decision making, 198–200
Controlled trials, randomized. See *Randomized controlled trial(s).*

Cost-effectiveness analysis, and viewpoint in economic evaluation, 286
   competing interventions and, 286–287
   methodologic considerations in, 291–294
   preconditions for, 286–287
   relevant treatment options and, 286
   use in plastic surgery clinical research, **285–296**
Cost-effectiveness plane, 288, 289
Craniofacial conditions, children with, questionnaire to measure quality of life issues in, 257–262
Craniofacial Youth Quality of Life Instrument-Craniofacial Surgery Module Youth Quality of Life Instrument-Facial Differences Module, 259

D

Decision analytic tree, 292
Decision making, surgical. See *Surgical decision making*.
Disabilities of the Arm and Shoulder questionnaire, 245
Dutch Burn Outcomes Questionnaire, 10–18 years adolescent form, 259
Dutch Health Outcomes Burn Questionnaire, 0–4 years parent form, 259
   5–18 years parent form, 259

E

Economic evaluations, in clinical practice, 294–295
   sensitivity analysis and, 294
   types of, 288–291
European Organization for Research and Treatment of Cancer (EORTC), Head and Neck (HN)-C35 Module, 232
   Quality of LIfe Questionnaire (QLQ) C30, 232, 233
Evidence-based plastic surgery, 203
Evidence pyramid, hierarchy of, 196

F

Functional Assessment of Cancer Therapy: Head and Neck (FACT-H&N), 232
Functional Assessment of Cancer Therapy (FACT): General (G), 232
Functional Living Index for Cancer (FLIC), 232

G

Gartland and Werley score, 245

H

Hand function, objective measures of, 241
   patient-reported measures of, 241–246
Hand outcomes, patient-reported, condition-specific insturument reommendations for, 246

Hand-related conditions, patient-reported outcome instruments for, 245
Hand surgery, economic burden of, 246–247
   measuring outcomes in, **239–250**
   outcomes research in, external funding for, 247
   future of, 247–248
HCUP Kids' Inpatient Database, 243
HCUP Nationwide Inpatient Database, 242
HCUP Nationwide Inpatient Sample, 242
HCUP State Ambulatory Surgery Database, 242
HCUP State Emergency Department Databases, 243
Head and neck, quality-of-life problems, solutions to, 234–235
   quality-of-life studies, problems and cautions in, 234
   reconstruction of, assessment of defect for, 230
      bilobed free osteocutaneous fibula flaps for, 229
      clinical research in, **227–237**
         quality-of-life instruments in, 231–234
         quality-of-life studies in, 231
      glossectomy and primary closure, 230
Health care databases, nationally available, 242–243
Health outcomes, patient-reported measures of, 241

I

Infant and toddler quality of life, 255

K

Karnofsky score, 232
KINDL, 255

L

Literature search, in systematic review, 210–211

M

Medical Outcomes Study Short Form 36 (SF-36), 232
Medicare Hospital Outpatient Standard Analytic File, 243
Medicare Physician/Supplier File, 243
Medicare Provider Analysis and Review File, 243
Michigan Hand Questionnaire, 245

N

Narrative reviews, in clinical research and practice, 208
National Surgical Quality Improvement Program, of the American College of Surgeons, 242
   of the Department of Veterans Affairs, 242

O

Osteocutaneous fibula flaps, bilobed free, for reconstruction of head and neck, 230

Outcome instruments, aesthetic surgery and, 272
Outcomes research, and assessment of quality of plans and providers, 239
    endpoint measures in, 239–240
    meta-analysis in, 241

P

Patient Evaluation Measure, 245
Patient Related Wrist Evaluation, 245
Pectus Excavaum Evaluation Questionnaire, 261, 262
Pediatric plastic surgery, clinical research in, and systematic review of quality-of-life questionnaires, **251–267**
    case-control studies in, 252
    case series in, 252
    cohort studies and, 252
    methodology in, 257
    randomized controlled trials in, 252–253
    study designs used in, 251–254
  outcome of, measurement of, 254–257
  quality-of-life instruments in, systematic review of, 257
  quality-of-life outcomes of, 254
  systematic reviews of, 253–254
  traditional outcome measures of, 254
Pediatric Voice Outcomes Survey, 261
Pediatric Voice-Related Quality-of-Life, 261
Performance Status Scale for Head and Neck (PSS-HN), 232
Plastic surgery, clinical research in, use of cost-effectiveness analysis in, **285–296**
  decision making in, factors in, 196
  evidence-based, 203
  new techniques in, 285
  randomized controlled trial in, role of, **275–284**
  techniques in, choice of, 285–286
    outcomes of, 286
Postmastectomy reconstruction, clinical research in breast surgery and, **215–226**

Q

Quality improvement interventions, benchmarking problem and, 299–301
  designs for, 300–301
  enumerative versus analytis studies in, 301
  error proofing/mistake proofing in, 301–302
  factorial experiments with multiple factors in, 301
  FOCUS-PDCA and, 298
  innovation in, 302
  PICOT and, 298–299
  reporting results of, 302
  safer health care and, 298
  saving five million lives and, 297–298
  saving one hundred thousand lives and, 297
  surgeons reporting errors and, 299
  testing quality of, **297–303**
Quality-of-life instruments, condition-specific measures, used in children treated by plastic surgeons, 258–261
  pediatric, generic, 255
Quality-of-life questionnaires, systematic review of, clinical research in pediatric plastic surgery, **251–267**
Quality-of-life studies, in clinical research in head and neck reconstruction, 231, 234

R

Randomized controlled trial(s), blinding in, 280–281
  concealment in, 279
  description of, 275
  differential care and, 278
  expertise-based study design in, 279–280
  importance of randomization in, 275–276
  in plastic surgery, design and execution of, challenges in, 277–282
    role of, **275–284**
  intention-to-treat analysis and, 281–282
  methods of randomization in, 278–279
  reporting of, 276
  state of surgical equipoise and, 277
  strategies for reducing loss to follow-up in, 280, 282
  strengths of, 276
  surgical learning curve and, 277–278
  treatment effect in, and implications to sample size, 282
Research question, clinical, reasons to pursue, 190
  clinically relevant, identification of, 189–190
  design of, feasibility of, 191
  final, formulation of, 191–193
  forming of, **189–193**
  formulation of, initial groundwork for, 190–191
  iterative research process and, 193
  plausibility of, 190
  resources available for project and, 191
  support from colleagues and, 191
  support within research group and, 189

S

SEER, 242
Study quality, evaluation of, in systematic review, 211–212
Surgical care, national trends in, 240
Surgical complications, assessment of, 240–241
Surgical decision making, basic science of, 201
  case reports and series in, 200–201
  cohort studies and case-controlled studies in, 198–200
  evidence-based clinical practice and, 195–196
  grading of evidence and, 202, 203
  hierarchy of evidence limitations and, 201–203

historical perspective on, 197
observational studies in, 198–200
physiologic studies for, 201
randomized controlled trials and, 197–198, 199
study design and hierarchy of evidence for, **195–205**
study designs for, properties of, 199
systemic reviews and meta-analyses and, 197
Surgical interventions, competing costs of,
  comparative analysis of, 287, 288
    discounting costs of, 291
    incremental cost-utility ratios and, 294
Surgical trials, blinding in evaluation of, 230
  cohort studies of, 229–231
  levels of evidence-research design rating in, 228
  methodologic challenges in, 227–228
  randomized controlled, surgical decision making and, 197–198, 199
  randomized trial and, 230–231
  study designs of, 228–229
Systematic review(s), data analysis and, 212
  data extraction form and, 212
  evaluation of study quality in, 211–212
  in clinical research and practice, **207–214**
  literature search in, 210–211
  research protocol in, 209–210
  research question and protocol of, 209
  results and interpretation of, 212–213
  steps in conducting, 209–213

T

Tacqol, 255
Trials, surgical. See *Surgical trials.*

U

University of Washington (UW) QOL, 232, 233
Upper Limb Functional Index, 245

Y

Youth quality of life instrument, 255